Learning Supportive Psychotherapy

An Illustrated Guide

Second Edition

T0176378

corecompetencies
in psychotherapy

Glen O. Gabbard, M.D., Series Editor

Learning Supportive Psychotherapy

An Illustrated Guide

Second Edition

Arnold Winston, M.D.
Chairman Emeritus, Department of Psychiatry and Behavioral Sciences, Mount Sinai Beth Israel, New York, New York; Professor Emeritus, Department of Psychiatry and Behavioral Sciences, Icahn School of Medicine at Mount Sinai, New York, New York; Professor and Associate Chairman, Department of Psychiatry, St. George's University School of Medicine, St. George's, Grenada

Richard N. Rosenthal, M.D., M.A.
Director of Addiction Psychiatry, Department of Psychiatry and Behavioral Health, Stony Brook Medicine, Stony Brook, New York; Professor of Psychiatry, Department of Psychiatry and Behavioral Health, Renaissance School of Medicine at Stony Brook University, Stony Brook, New York; Adjunct Professor of Psychiatry, Icahn School of Medicine at Mount Sinai, New York, New York

Laura Weiss Roberts, M.D., M.A.
Chairman and Katharine Dexter McCormick and Stanley McCormick Memorial Professor, Department of Psychiatry and Behavioral Sciences, Stanford University School of Medicine, Stanford, California

AMERICAN
PSYCHIATRIC
ASSOCIATION
PUBLISHING

Disclosures of interests: The authors have no competing interests or conflicts to declare.

If you wish to buy 50 or more copies of the same title, please go to www.appi.org/special discounts for more information.

American Psychiatric Association Publishing
800 Maine Avenue SW
Suite 900
Washington, DC 20024-2812
www.appi.org

Library of Congress Cataloging-in-Publication Data
Names: Winston, Arnold, 1935– author. | Rosenthal, Richard N., author. | Roberts, Laura Weiss, 1960– author. | American Psychiatric Association Publishing, issuing body.
Title: Learning supportive psychotherapy : an illustrated guide / by Arnold Winston, Richard N. Rosenthal, Laura Weiss Roberts.
Other titles: Core competencies in psychotherapy.
Description: Second edition. | Washington, D.C. : American Psychiatric Association Publishing, [2020] | Series: Core competencies in psychotherapy | Includes bibliographical references and index. |
Identifiers: LCCN 2019037391 (print) | LCCN 2019037392 (ebook) | ISBN 9781615372348 (paperback ; alk. paper) | ISBN 9781615372874 (ebook)
Subjects: MESH: Psychotherapy—methods | Professional-Patient Relations | Psychotherapeutic Processes
Classification: LCC RC480.5 (print) | LCC RC480.5 (ebook) | NLM WM 420 | DDC 616.89/14—dc23
LC record available at https://lccn.loc.gov/2019037391
LC ebook record available at https://lccn.loc.gov/2019037392

British Library Cataloguing in Publication Data
A CIP record is available from the British Library.

Contents

Introduction

We are pleased to present a revised edition of our book, *Learning Supportive Psychotherapy*, first published in 2004 as *Introduction to Supportive Psychotherapy* and revised in 2012. One of our authors, Dr. Henry Pinsker, has retired, but we have been fortunate to find an outstanding new coauthor, Dr. Laura Roberts, who brings a wealth of experience and expertise to this new edition.

This book is written for beginning therapists who need to learn the fundamentals of psychotherapy and in particular need to learn how to talk with psychotherapy patients. All practitioners search for effective ways to treat patients. We believe that the beginning resident attempting to practice supportive psychotherapy needs clear guidelines for the conduct and progression of psychotherapy from beginning to end. Accordingly, we have attempted to present straightforward guidelines to help the beginner in four major areas:

- Forming and maintaining a positive therapeutic alliance
- Understanding and formulating patients' problems
- Setting realistic treatment goals
- Knowing what to say to patients (technique)

After introducing the concept of supportive psychotherapy, we present the basic principles of this treatment approach and the position of supportive psychotherapy on a continuum from supportive to expressive psychotherapy on the basis of the extent and level of a patient's psychopathology. We describe supportive psychotherapy interventions available to the therapist, the process of performing a thorough patient evaluation and case formulation, and the process of setting realistic goals with the patient. The general framework of supportive psychotherapy—including indications, phases of treatment, initiation and termination of sessions, and professional boundaries—is outlined. We include therapeutic relationship issues (transference, countertransference, therapeutic alliance) and self-disclosure guidelines.

We then discuss crisis intervention, which uses many supportive psychotherapy approaches, and the applicability of supportive psychotherapy to special populations, including patients with chronic mental illness, substance use disorders, and co-occurring conditions. We conclude the book with a discussion of how to determine whether a psychiatry resident has achieved competence in supportive psychotherapy and with a presentation of the evidence for the efficacy of supportive psychotherapy, including a number of outcome trials. The final chapter includes a number of questions for self-study.

Arnold Winston, M.D.
Richard N. Rosenthal, M.D., M.A.
Laura Weiss Roberts, M.D., M.A.

Acknowledgments

Residents at Beth Israel Medical Center and St. Luke's-Roosevelt Hospital Center were recruited as patients and therapists for the psychotherapy videos. We are grateful for their efforts in production of these videos. The following residents participated from Beth Israel Medical Center: Caroline Blackman, M.D., Nivea Calico, M.D., David Edgcomb, M.D., and Glenn Occhiogrosso, M.D. The following residents participated from St. Luke's-Roosevelt Hospital Center: Justin Capote, M.D., Nonso Ekene Enekwechi, M.D., Adrienne Mishkin, M.D., and Vinod Pachagiri Suresh, M.D.

We wish to acknowledge the importance of the Beth Israel Brief Psychotherapy Research Program in providing the milieu for the writing of this book and our appreciation of our colleagues from this program, especially John Christopher Muran, Jeremy Safran, and Lisa Wallner Samstag. Finally, we are grateful to the Supportive Psychotherapy Study Group, including Victor Goldin, Esther Goldman, David Hellerstein, David Janeway, Steve Klee, Lee Shomstein, Fran Silverman, Jeffrey Solgan, Adam Wilensky, and Philip Yanowitch, for help in developing many of the ideas contained in this book.

We also wish to express our appreciation to Gabrielle Termuehlen, Tenzin Tsungmey, and Ann Tennier for their excellent work in editing, engaging with the authors, and performing literature reviews in the development of this most recent edition.

Video Guide

The videos in this book provide detailed examples of supportive psychotherapy. Each video includes text boxes at the bottom of the screen highlighting the therapist's interventions. The videos can be viewed online by navigating to **www.appi.org/Winston** and using the embedded video player. The videos are optimized for most current operating systems, including mobile operating systems.

> ▶ **Video cues provided in the text identify the vignette by title and approximate run time.**

Case Vignettes

Chapter 3. Assessment, Case Formulation, and Goal Setting

Vignette 1: Assessment (9:54)

This vignette illustrates how to perform a thorough assessment of a new patient while developing and maintaining a therapeutic alliance.

Chapter 4. Techniques

Vignette 2: Severe, Persistent Mental Illness in an Uncooperative Patient (13:42)

This vignette illustrates a highly supportive approach with an uncooperative patient who has a great deal of psychopathology.

Vignette 3: Supportive-Expressive Treatment (30:49)

This vignette is of a reasonably well integrated young woman who is treated with supportive-expressive psychotherapy.

Chapter 5. General Framework of Supportive Psychotherapy

Vignette 4: Addressing a Misalliance (6:22)

In this vignette, the therapist addresses a misalliance within the patient-therapist relationship and "owns up" to making a mistake, which helps to alleviate the misalliance.

Chapter 7. Crisis Intervention

Vignette 5: Crisis Intervention (18:00)

This vignette illustrates a number of different techniques that can be used for a patient with posttraumatic stress disorder.

> *Session 1 (0:00–7:13)*
> *Session 2 (7:14–12:47)*
> *Session 4 (12:48–15:03)*
> *Session 5 (15:04–18:00)*

Chapter 8. Applicability to Special Populations

Vignette 6: Substance Use Disorder (7:00)

This vignette illustrates the use of psychoeducation in a patient with substance use disorder in order to address the patient's use of denial and the moral model of addiction.

Evolution of the Concept of Supportive Psychotherapy

1

Origins

Supportive psychotherapy is a treatment approach focused on patients' overall health and well-being and their abilities to adapt constructively to their life circumstances. The domain of supportive psychotherapy has become larger in recent years, reflecting changes in the definition, and even more so in the practice, of psychotherapy. Today, supportive psychotherapy has a robust evidence base and plays an important role in the care of individuals living with diverse mental and physical disorders and in the care of individuals facing difficult life events or experiences, such as the transition to college, the birth of a child, changes in employment, divorce, and bereavement.

Supportive psychotherapy was developed in the early twentieth century as a treatment approach with more limited objectives than psychoanalysis, which had previously been the only psychological treatment in medicine. Psychoanalysis and psychotherapy were originally developed as treatments for *neurosis*, which was the principal concern of office-based (i.e., nonhospital) psychiatrists. Neurosis was conceptualized as an unconscious attempt to solve a psychological conflict. As psychotherapy became more widely accepted, therapists applied psychotherapeutic techniques to a broad range of problems that were outside the scope of the earliest psychotherapy and not adequately explained by the theories associated with it. Because of practical considerations, including affordability, a course of treatment often consisted of a small number of visits, and the objective was limited to relief of the presenting problem. Therapists found it necessary to be more interactive and responsive with patients. Flexible response to clinical reality called for more general use of supportive approaches. Although some therapists feared that they were diluting "real" psychotherapy by not adhering to its rules, therapists were, in fact, applying a different psychotherapy.

Psychoanalytic thinkers who formulated theories about the causes of symptoms and personality problems created a general theory of mental organization and behavior referred to as *psychodynamic theory*. Many concepts of psychodynamic theory have become so widely disseminated that they are now accepted as established truths about mental life by much of the educated public in the Western world. Therapy that was not psychoanalysis but that instead was based on theories developed by psychoanalysts became known as *psychodynamic psychotherapy*. This therapy has been called psychoanalytically oriented psychotherapy, intensive psychotherapy, uncovering psychotherapy, change-oriented psychotherapy, insight-directed psychotherapy, or—the term we employ—*expressive psychotherapy* (not to be confused with dance therapy, art therapy, and so forth, which have also been designated as "expressive").

Between 1950 and 1970, psychodynamic psychotherapy became the most widely practiced psychological treatment approach in the United States. It was taught as the embodiment of theories of personality development, with the objectives of reversing the primary disease process or restructuring the personality (Ursano and Silberman 1999).

Although *personality change* is invariably assumed to be the objective in the psychotherapy literature, for many patients, the objective is stability and adaptation, not fundamental change. The objectives of supportive treatment, as initially defined, were not to change a patient's personality but rather to help a patient cope with symptoms, to prevent relapse of a serious mental illness, or to help a relatively healthy person deal with a transient problem. Supportive psychotherapy differed from traditional psychoanalytic treatment in that the therapist played an active and direct role in the therapeutic relationship.

Authors continue to propose different definitions of supportive psychotherapy (Douglas 2008; Winston et al. 1986) and continue to hold different opinions about whether or not supportive psychotherapy is a psychodynamic therapy or a distinctive form of therapy. The problem of definition is compounded by the coexistence of two incompatible definitions of psychodynamic therapy. Some writers use the term *psychodynamic psychotherapy* broadly to describe any therapy in which the therapist's *understanding* of mental life is based on theories developed by psychoanalytic writers; other authors use the term narrowly to describe only therapies that employ the essential *techniques* of expressive therapy.

Definitions of supportive psychotherapy have been organized around four themes:

1. What the therapist hopes to achieve (objectives)—for example, to maintain or improve the patient's self-esteem, to minimize or prevent recurrence of symptoms, and to maximize the patient's adaptive capacities (Pinsker et al. 1991)
2. What the patient wants to achieve (goals)—for example, to maintain or reestablish the patient's best possible level of functioning given the limitations of his or her personality, inherent ability, and life circumstances (Ursano and Silberman 1999)
3. What the therapist does (technique)—for example, encouragement, reassurance, education, and advice
4. What it is not—that is, an exposition of elements that have been subtracted from expressive therapy (Dewald 1964, 1971)

In addressing the question of where supportive psychotherapy fits among the many models of psychotherapy, Rockland (1989) proposed the acronym POST to signify *psychodynamically oriented supportive therapy*, explaining that all psychotherapies involve both supportive and exploratory interventions and that therapy should be "based on as complete an understanding as possible of the patient's core conflicts, characteristic defensive maneuvers, ego functions, superego organization, and object relations" (p. 7). Although Rockland's acronym has not caught on, his thinking reflects the views of most people who have written about supportive psychotherapy in the past 25 years.

A therapist who accepts the following tenets of modern psychodynamic therapy is a psychodynamically oriented therapist (Fonagy and Target 2009):

- Assumption of psychological causation
- Assumption of limitations of consciousness and the influence of unconscious mental states
- Assumption of internal representations of interpersonal relationships
- Assumption of ubiquity of psychological conflict

- Assumption of psychic defenses
- Assumption of complex meaning
- Assumption of emphasis on the therapeutic relationship
- Assumption of the validity of a developmental perspective

According to Gabbard (2017, pp. 4–18), three elements of psychodynamic psychotherapy pertain to the therapist's understanding of the patient:

- Much of mental life is unconscious.
- Childhood experiences in concert with genetic factors shape the adult.
- Symptoms and behaviors serve multiple functions and are determined by complex and often unconscious forces.

Three elements of psychodynamic psychotherapy pertain to the therapist's actions, or to the conduct of the treatment:

- The patient's transference to the therapist is a primary source of understanding.
- The therapist's countertransference provides valuable understanding about what the patient induces in others.
- The patient's resistance to the therapeutic process is a major focus of the therapy.

A final element of psychodynamic psychotherapy describes the objective, or what the therapist hopes to accomplish:

- The goal is to assist the patient in achieving a sense of authenticity and uniqueness.

The psychodynamically oriented therapist practicing supportive psychotherapy understands the patient in terms of the first three of Gabbard's (2017) points but does not conduct treatment in the manner described in the next three points. Transference is used only to the extent necessary. *Resistance* might be used without implications about unconscious process to describe the patient's clinging to familiar patterns. Although the therapist would be pleased to achieve the outcome described in the last point, the formal objectives of supportive psychotherapy are limited to symptom relief and better adaptation in promoting overall health and personal well-being.

The early characterization of supportive psychotherapy as a limited approach was based on its deviation from classical theory. Although the rationale and techniques of today's supportive psychotherapy can be explained in terms of theory, the techniques were developed from practical work with patients. Novalis et al. (1993, p. 5) observed, "Virtually all of the several hundred psychotherapies are based upon a concept or theory of mind. Supportive psychotherapy…is not dependent upon any specific overriding concept or theory, but utilizes the rich work done by many theorists in understanding how people change as this work is confirmed empirically."

Psychodynamic Therapy and the Supportive-Expressive Continuum

In his textbook *Psychotherapy: A Dynamic Approach*, Dewald (1971) explained the contrast between supportive psychotherapy and insight-directed therapy (i.e., expressive therapy, in our terminology), observing that a patient's treatment usually falls somewhere in between the two (Figure 1–1). As Dewald (1964) noted, "The ends of the continuum can be clearly distinguished from each other in regards to the theory of psychotherapy, and to the technique which evolves logically from this theory. In the center of the continuum these differences are less discrete and less clearly demarcated. The treatment of most patients involves both supportive and expressive elements, which must be used in a coherent, integrated fashion" (p. 97).

Dewald described supportive psychotherapy as generally aimed at symptom relief and overt behavior change, without emphasis on modifying personality or resolving unconscious conflict. He wrote, "The majority of people with psychiatric illness…, character problems, acute or chronic psychosis, etc., are not suitable candidates for a formal attempt at insight-directed psychotherapy. Instead they are more suitably and expeditiously treated by a dynamically oriented supportive approach" (Dewald 1971, p. 114).

Expressive therapy is a collective term for a variety of approaches that seek personality change through analysis of the relationship between the therapist and patient and through the acquisition of insight about previously unrecognized feelings, thoughts, needs, and conflicts, which the patient must attempt to consciously resolve and better integrate. We prefer using the term expressive therapy in order to avoid using the word *psychodynamic* with two different meanings.

To emphasize that the treatment of each patient involves both supportive and expressive elements, a linear representation of this continuum has been presented by a number of authors (see Figure 1–1). At one end, the frequency of supportive interventions is high and the frequency of exploratory intervention is low. At the other end, the frequency of supportive interventions is low. The supportive and expressive *stances*, or points of view, are very different. The most supportive stance involves guidance, whereas

| Supportive relationship | Counseling | Supportive psychotherapy | Supportive-expressive psychotherapy | Expressive-supportive psychotherapy | Psychoanalysis |

Figure 1–1.   Supportive-expressive continuum.

the most expressive stance involves discovery. Luborsky and Mark (1991, p. 110) described expressive therapies as "techniques aimed at facilitating the patient's expressions about problems and conflicts and their understanding." The supportive position may encourage use of a defense; the expressive position may seek to discover the roots of the defense with the hope that its use will end. Even though treatment invariably entails both supportive and expressive elements, the therapist's basic stance, at a single point in treatment of a patient, must be primarily one or the other. When the stance is expressive, the therapist follows the dictum "be as expressive as you can be, and as supportive as you have to be" (Wallerstein 1986, p. 688). When the stance is supportive, the therapist follows Wachtel's (1993) advice: "Be as supportive as you can be so that you can be as expressive as you will need to be" (p. 155). This distinction is critical.

If asked what they are doing, most practitioners will respond "psychotherapy" or "supportive psychotherapy" or "psychoanalytically oriented psychotherapy" or "psychodynamic psychotherapy." It is important to note that the world of psychotherapy has changed greatly, and psychotherapy is no longer limited to approaches based on psychodynamic formulations. Supportive interventions may be used productively in the conduct of cognitive-behavioral therapy, for example, without raising significant theoretical or practical problems. The graphic representation in Figure 1–1 is not an indication that the patient population is distributed on a bell-shaped curve. Essentially, when we describe the conceptual basis of therapy, supportive-expressive psychotherapy and expressive-supportive psychotherapy meet at the center of the visual representation. When we describe practical work with patients, we believe that supportive-expressive psychotherapy is what most practitioners are doing most of the time with most of their patients.

If the treatment of each patient involves both supportive and expressive elements, why are the elements taught separately? As Rockland (1989) pointed out, "supportive and exploratory psychotherapies…[are] sufficiently discrepant in major ways to deserve clear differentiation and separation" (p. 20). Supportive psychotherapy, expressive therapy, cognitive-behavioral therapy, family therapy, and group therapy, among others, are all taught by different specialists because there is a lot to know about each of them. As in all areas of education, it is the task of the student to integrate all that he or she has learned.

We appreciate that many, many approaches to therapy have been named that emphasize an element of treatment, personality development, or symptom formation that is thought to be novel or especially significant. Although, as Winston and Winston (2002) said, theories "are described separately to maintain clarity, these various models come together to inform the psychotherapy approach for a given patient" (p. 13).

"Therapists…should be able to transition from one approach to another. Such transitioning involves combining various interventions from different psychotherapy traditions into a cohesive therapy" (p. 264).

Definition of Supportive Psychotherapy

The term *supportive therapy* is frequently used in nonpsychiatric studies to denote an approach that involves expression of interest, attention to concrete services, encouragement, and optimism. This is a supportive *relationship* or supportive *contact* but not supportive *psychotherapy*. Supportive relationships with family, friends, coworkers, clergy, and others may indeed be useful and sustaining, but in our opinion they should not be called "therapy." We note, too, that the boundary between counseling and psychotherapy is not clear. Supportive psychotherapy is based on diagnostic evaluation; the therapist's actions are deliberate and designed to achieve specified objectives. The professional relationship is unique and exists solely to meet the needs of the patient. The therapist's gratification must come from doing the job well, rather than from the patient's expressions of gratitude or from using the patient as an audience. In everyday life, there are many motivations for being supportive. In the professional supportive relationship, the motivation must be to meet the patient's needs—to help the patient adapt and cope in order to live his or her best life.

In psychiatric literature, the terms supportive therapy and supportive psychotherapy have been used interchangeably. This is unfortunate because the nonspecific support provided to patients who have medical or surgical problems is also characterized as supportive therapy, in this case referring to efforts that make the patient more comfortable. We will always use the long form—supportive psychotherapy—to emphasize that we are writing about a professional service that is provided in a mental health context by a person trained in mental health theory and practices.

We define *supportive psychotherapy* as a dyadic treatment that uses direct techniques to 1) ameliorate symptoms and 2) maintain, restore, or improve self-esteem, ego function, and adaptive skills (see below) with a focus on the patient's overall health and well-being. Treatment may examine real or transferential relationships and past and current patterns of emotional response or behavior in order to accomplish these objectives.

- *Self-esteem* involves the patient's sense of efficacy, confidence, hope, and self-regard.
- *Ego functions* include relation to reality, thinking, defense formation, regulation of affect, synthetic function, and others, as enumerated by

Beres (1956, pp. 164–235), Bellak (1958, pp. 1–40), and other authors. Ego functions could alternatively be called *psychological functions* because they are addressed by behavior therapists and cognitive therapists whose formulations do not include the ego as a component of a mental apparatus. Ego functions are often categorized as psychic structure. As cognitive functions are increasingly understood in physical and physiological terms, psychological terminology may be eclipsed, but it still appears to be useful in the clinical setting at present.

- *Adaptive skills* are actions associated with effective functioning. Social skills are one example of an adaptive skill for individuals living with a chronic psychotic disorder or personality disorder. The boundary between ego functions and adaptive skills is not sharply defined. The patient's assessment of events is an ego function; the action taken in response to the assessment is an adaptive skill.

We have explained that supportive and expressive therapies are different and that the treatment of an individual patient is likely to involve elements of both. In practice, *supportive psychotherapy*, as we have defined it, describes what is identified as supportive-expressive psychotherapy on the continuum. When we teach or prescribe psychodynamic therapy, we are usually referring to what is identified on the continuum as expressive-supportive psychotherapy. Most psychotherapists in the United States are guided by psychodynamic principles, but it is possible to address self-esteem issues, ego-function problems, and adaptive skills without accepting psychodynamic principles.

In the following three examples, the therapists' approaches represent different points along the supportive-expressive continuum.

Case Illustration 1

Juan is a 55-year-old man who attended school for 6 years in his native country in Latin America. In the United States, he has held various unskilled jobs. He was married for several years, but his wife divorced him when he became involved with illicit substances. He has been drug-free since serving a 2-year prison sentence 20 years ago, but he has had increased difficulty obtaining work. He now has several medical problems, and he keeps his clinic appointments and follows prescribed treatment. A resident has monitored his antidepressant medication in the psychiatric clinic once a month for more than a year. Juan attends a day program for medical patients, but he has been threatened with expulsion because he is quick to show anger and lash out if he feels that someone is pushing him aside at lunchtime or taking the seat he wished to occupy. The day program and his clinic visits are his only structured activity. The treating resident discusses the recommendations of the other physicians with Juan and talks about the effects of his medications, encouraging Juan to tell the other physicians if he has any problems. The resident responds empathically to Juan's descriptions of loneliness and praises Juan for his success at maintaining sobriety. The resident is satisfied that Juan's angry responses are not associated with delusional thinking, but she has been unable to involve Juan in scrutinizing the reason for his angry responses or offering anything but the most superficial justifications for his actions. Juan does accept the suggestion that he should always seek help from a staff member if he is angered by other participants in the day program. *(This is an entirely supportive approach, involving encouragement, praise, and advice about adaptive skills. Success will be measured by the patient's continued acceptance of medical treatment and antidepressant medication and ability to control his temper.)*

Case Illustration 2

Richard has the same problems as Juan, but he has a greater ability to think about his internal life. He says that if someone gets ahead of him, he feels that the person is putting him down and mocking him. Richard says he was brought up this way. When he did not stand up for himself, his father would become very angry and punish him, and no one in his family or neighborhood would have considered his father to be wrong. The therapist explains that people with such experiences in the past may be quick to defend themselves from what appears to be an affront, and Richard agrees that this makes sense. *(The therapy in this case is supportive-expressive because it involves assumptions about mental life. The therapist seeks to help the patient begin to understand problem-causing behavior in terms of attitudes about which he had been unaware.)*

Case Illustration 3

George is aware of having an "anger problem" and becomes very irritable when his therapist asks, as he had done in previous sessions, whether George has been involved in any conflicts since the last visit. George responds sullenly and tells the therapist that the medication he had been taking for several months was causing too many side effects and wasn't helping at all. The therapist suggests that perhaps being asked about possible failures of self-control reminds George of his childhood experience of being scolded by his father. George says he hadn't thought of that, but it might be true. *(Suspecting that the patient's anger might be of transferential origin, the therapist suggests a link between past and present relationships—an expressive element. This therapy may be described as located at the midpoint of the supportive-expressive continuum.)*

Teaching Supportive Psychotherapy

Although supportive psychotherapy is the most widely practiced form of psychodynamically oriented psychotherapy, teaching supportive psychotherapy poses challenges. Supportive psychotherapy is not based on rigorous and internally consistent or appealing theory, and it does not offer solutions to intractable clinical problems. The field has no conferences, no stars, and relatively few books.

Education of psychotherapists throughout much of the twentieth century was based primarily on principles developed by psychoanalysts. In a short text for beginners, Balsam and Balsam (1984) wrote, "The psychotherapist's central task is learning to understand…the emotional experience of the patient" (p. 1). Treatment techniques that had specific rationales in psychoanalysis were presented as universal techniques required for *all* psychotherapy. If the patient stopped talking, the therapist was advised to wait for him or her to continue or to ask what he or she was thinking. The therapist was advised to avoid direct answers to questions (Colby 1951, pp. 55–56). In short, the treatment that was taught was intended "to relieve the patient of distressing neurotic symptoms or discordant personality characteristics" (Colby 1951, p. 3).

This model provided no guidance about how to work with patients who were inarticulate or poorly educated, patients who had intractable social problems or severe behavioral problems, or patients who were expected to drop out after a few monthly or bimonthly visits. Psychotherapists who failed to discover how to conduct supportive psychotherapy provided their patients an irrational, unintegrated mixture of expressive assumptions and supportive tactics.

In a recent review, Brenner (2012) advocated for a much more sophisticated approach to teaching supportive psychotherapy in the twenty-first century. He suggested that the mandate for competence in supportive psychotherapy, the strong evidence base for supportive psychotherapy, and the growing prominence of the recovery movement in psychiatry all served to demonstrate the importance of greater curricular attention to supportive psychotherapy in psychiatric residency programs. Brenner articulated three important factors in teaching supportive psychotherapy: its relevance for common factors underlying all forms of psychotherapy; its role on a spectrum of psychodynamically informed psychotherapies; and its value as a modality that includes specifically definable techniques and aims. Brenner highlighted several examples of the importance of supportive psychotherapy, including helping patients with emotional regulation, grief, impulsivity, reality-testing, self-esteem, responsibility-taking, and healthy self-identification. Moreover, Brenner recommended teaching supportive psychotherapy in diverse clinical rotations, including inpatient and consultation-liaison services as well as ambulatory settings.

In time, residents who have received training in supportive psychotherapy will observe that patients with the greatest psychological strengths are suitable for treatment that is primarily expressive. Nevertheless, the fact that a patient has the resources and psychological characteristics needed to undergo expressive therapy does not mean that expressive therapy is indicated. Providing more support than needed may be effective but may deprive the patient of an opportunity to make more impressive changes in his or her life. As Hellerstein et al. (1994) pointed out, a strong case can be made for employing the supportive (i.e., supportive-expressive) model for most patients, shifting to more time-intensive expressive measures only to the extent required. In all cases, treatment planning must involve consideration of what the patient wants to accomplish.

Supervisors working with residents may note that the fundamental objectives of supportive psychotherapy can be achieved by early career clinicians who may not have much exposure to psychodynamic principles. Beginners who cannot yet attempt expressive psychotherapy may be competent at providing good supportive-expressive treatment. With practice, therapists become aware of how a patient is responding to them and then of how they are responding to the patient. Viederman (2008) described a very active approach in which the clinician asks the patient for memories about earlier times in life that are related to the clinician's observations and interpretations and then communicates to the patient an understanding of the patient's predicament. He wrote, "The consultant enters the patient's world, develops a picture of him, of his experience with people in his life, and communicates this in a language which is familiar to him. This results in a climate that is the essence of a supportive relationship" (p. 352). One of the many satisfactions of being a psychotherapist is that the clinician improves and continues to improve as the decades pass. Supervisors working with residents who are learning supportive psychotherapy approaches may help establish the groundwork for such professional growth.

Conclusion

Supportive psychotherapy and the expressive psychotherapies have different objectives and employ different techniques. The treatment of an individual patient whose treatment plan calls for psychodynamically oriented supportive psychotherapy involves both supportive and expressive elements. The clinician must understand and must be able to integrate both approaches. Psychiatric residency programs must ensure that their graduates are competent in psychotherapeutic approaches, including supportive psychotherapy. Learning supportive psychotherapy can help reinforce the common factors underlying all forms of psychotherapy, aspects of psychodynamically informed psychotherapy, and specifically definable techniques and aims of psychotherapy.

Principles and Mode of Action

2

Underlying Assumptions

Supportive psychotherapy relies on *direct measures*. The therapist is active and addresses conscious problems or conflicts rather than underlying unconscious conflicts or personality distortions (Dewald 1994). A major tenet of Freud's early psychoanalytic work was that symptoms are caused by unconscious conflict; through psychoanalysis, the conflict becomes conscious and is worked through, and then the symptoms disappear because they are no longer psychologically necessary. In supportive psychotherapy, it is not assumed that improvement will develop as a by-product of insight. Greater self-awareness or insight about the origin of problems is not essential.

In supportive therapy, the *relationship* between patient and therapist is a relationship between two adults with a common purpose. As in all professional relationships, one person provides a service that the other requires. The professional person, the therapist, owes the patient respect, full attention, honesty, and vigorous effort to accomplish the stated purpose by using the knowledge and skills of the profession. Adhering to these obligations is known as staying within boundaries. Because the therapist is understood to be a whole person, with professional training and life experience, and is not required to be minimally communicative or to be a "blank slate" in the therapeutic relationship, there is greater symmetry between the patient and therapist than in other therapeutic relationships.

This said, the relationship in supportive psychotherapy is wholly focused on fostering the overall health and well-being of the patient, on reducing symptoms and sources of distress, and on bolstering his or her adaptive strengths. The interaction may be friendly, but the two individuals do not become friends. The therapist does not advise the patient on how to vote, whom to marry, or how to decorate the home. The therapist does not seek assistance from the patient. If the therapist talks at length, describing his or her own experiences, thoughts, or feelings, the therapist must consider whether it is really for the patient's benefit or whether it is because the therapist enjoys talking. Using the patient in this manner is exploitation.

When the stance is expressive, the therapist tries to remain neutral and cautious when responding so that the patient's perception of thoughts and feelings about the therapist can be analyzed as projections of feelings associated with important figures in past or present life. This projection is termed *transference.* The expressive stance avoids responses that might encourage the patient to perceive the therapist as a person with opinions, tastes, family, or even personality. It is this technical maneuver that has produced the image of the psychotherapist as an individual who parries all questions with evasive answers or reflects all questions back to the patient.

The degree to which the therapist and patient discuss transference depends on the type of therapy. In expressive therapies, analysis of transference is a key element in the process of understanding the patient's inner life. Although transference occurs in supportive psychotherapy, as it does in all relationships, it is typically discussed only when manifestations of transference threaten the continuation of therapy. Because most psychotherapy is supportive-expressive in practice, transference is not a taboo subject. In relational therapies, which have been increasingly popular since the 1980s (Fonagy and Target 2009; Greenberg 2001; Mitchell 1988), intense and ongoing examination of the patient-therapist interaction is a major focus of the therapeutic process, and the therapist may disclose much more than would be done in classical treatment. This is not an approach to be undertaken by the novice therapist. Even at the supportive end of the spectrum, it is often useful for the therapist to try to make the patient aware of problems in their real-time interaction.

THERAPIST 1: You haven't said you disagree with me, but you have found something of concern with every observation I have made today *(a clarification that might encourage the patient to be more frank, without examining underlying issues)*.

THERAPIST 2: Are you aware that when I have tried to focus on steps you might take to manage better in daily life, you go back to talking about what your wife did wrong? *(an observation in the course of supportive-expressive therapy)*

THERAPIST 3: Are you aware that when I ask you about your father, you talk about problems at work or the world situation? *(confrontation in the course of expressive-supportive therapy)*

As stated earlier in this chapter, the supportive psychotherapy relationship is a relationship between two adults with a common purpose. The therapist encourages the development of positive feelings; if the patient brings up the presence of these positive feelings, the therapist accepts them without attempting to have the patient understand them. The patient's positive feelings about the therapist, even if moderately unrealistic, are useful for maintaining the therapeutic alliance and potentially useful for identification with the therapist. (For further discussion of the patient-therapist relationship, see Chapter 6, "The Therapeutic Relationship.")

PATIENT 1: You always have such a clear way of thinking about things. I'm all over the place. You always know what the problem is and what to do about it.

THERAPIST 1: Thanks. It's easier when you hear a description of a complex issue than when you're in the midst of it.

If negative feelings about the therapist or the therapy are evident, or even suspected, they must be discussed because negative feelings may threaten or lead to disruption of treatment.

PATIENT 2: Getting here seems to be more difficult. Things always come up at the last minute. I apologize for being late.

THERAPIST 2: We could try to change your appointment time if that would help, but I wonder if you're finding it more difficult now because you're having some doubts about continuing.

In expressive psychotherapy, the patient's reaction to events in his or her current life may be discussed as possible (unconscious) expressions of the patient's feelings about the therapist.

PATIENT: I was on the phone with customer service for half an hour. This really drives me up the wall. It was worse than ever. Those people are incompetent. I keep losing my temper.

THERAPIST: Last week you were complaining because I hadn't come up with a quick answer for all your problems. Maybe you were especially angry with customer service and saw them as incompetent because you were thinking I was incompetent and you were angry with me.

In supportive psychotherapy, however, events in the therapy may be offered as illustrations or models for everyday life.

PATIENT: This really drives me up the wall. It was worse than ever. Those people are incompetent. I keep losing my temper.

THERAPIST: Last week you were complaining because I hadn't come up with a quick answer for all your problems. You were polite and thoughtful, and we were able to discuss it, and you didn't seem to be "up the wall." Maybe you could be as reasonable and controlled when you talk to customer service as you are here with me.

In the course of supportive psychotherapy and supportive-expressive therapy, the therapist gives simple, direct answers to personal questions, within the bounds of information that he or she is willing to share with an acquaintance. The disclosure of information that is ordinarily kept private is often associated with a violation of the boundary that must separate the personal from the professional. These are nuanced judgments in the course of supportive psychotherapy— for example, a patient who recently moved from another state may inquire about the therapist's past moves after graduating from residency and moving to a new community. The therapist must decide whether responding with personal information will serve the therapeutic alliance and the goals of the therapeutic work or whether it will introduce complex transferential issues that are counter to the goals of treatment. When the stance is primarily expressive, the therapeutic strategy is based on the assumption that the patient's thoughts about the therapist will reveal evidence of transference. In supportive psychotherapy, the transferential aspect may be more or less relevant in relation to the goals of treatment.

Conversational Style

Supportive psychotherapy is conducted in a conversational style. Because conversation is the principal form of interaction among adults, readers might wonder why it is necessary for us to say anything about it in this book. When we first wrote about supportive psychotherapy, it was important to convey to the beginner that the therapist's task is not listening silently to a patient who has been instructed to "say whatever comes to mind." Today, the psychiatry resident who listens silently at length usually does so because he or she does not know what to say, or expects the patient to pause at any moment, or hopes that the next sentence will be important and that the patient will soon get to the point. The beginning therapist probably knows that by interrupting a silence too quickly, he or she may never know what is troubling the patient. When the therapeutic stance is supportive, the therapist will not wait long. Faced with a long pause, the expressive therapist thinks, "Is there an indication for me to speak?" In contrast, the supportive therapist thinks, "Is there a reason for me *not* to speak?"

The therapeutic interaction is conversational in style, but it is not normal conversation. In normal conversation, the speakers alternate: your turn, my turn. You tell me what happened on your way to work this morning, and I tell you what happened to me on my way to work; you talk about your pets, and I talk about my pets. In therapy, the therapist is *responsive*, but it is always the patient's turn.

Physicians who are new to psychotherapy often have had years of practice polishing a style of communication that is not responsive and not supportive. They have mastered the art of obtaining the history by asking questions. When every utterance is a question, the process is interrogation. Miller and Rollnick (1991, p. 66), writing about motivational interviewing, advised that one should not ask more than three questions in a row because doing so implies an interaction between an active expert and a passive patient. To maintain a supportive conversational style, the therapist must be responsive. In the act of responding, the therapist is giving something to the patient. Except for narcissistic individuals who get satisfaction from having an audience, people want to be given something in return for what they give, and this giving, by an intelligent, interested person—the therapist—is gratifying and reassuring.

To maintain a conversational style, the therapist responds both to what the patient volunteers and to the patient's responses to questions. Compare the following two interactions:

PATIENT 1: I slept better most of the time.
THERAPIST 1: OK.
PATIENT 1: But it's still hard being out of work; I'm just getting by on my unemployment checks.
THERAPIST 1: OK.
PATIENT 1: I try to keep busy, like you said.
THERAPIST 1: OK.
PATIENT 1: But I still feel bad some of the time.
THERAPIST 1: OK. *(This is a dreadful, nongiving style of response, not unusual in hospitals.)*

PATIENT 2: I slept better most of the time.
THERAPIST 2: I'm glad to hear it. And that's without medication, isn't it?
PATIENT 2: Yes. But it's still hard being out of work; I'm just getting by on my unemployment checks.
THERAPIST 2: When you are used to working, unemployment insurance is important, but it doesn't fill your life.
PATIENT 2: I try to keep busy, like you said.
THERAPIST 2: Good. What are you doing?
PATIENT 2: I've been cleaning my basement, bit by bit. Not just the floor, but cleaning the old grit from overhead pipes and things like that. It's not really important.
THERAPIST 2: It sounds like a project that isn't exciting, but you can see the results of what you have done.

PATIENT 2: But I still feel bad some of the time.
THERAPIST 2: I'm sorry to hear it. We have to work on that. *(The therapist's responses, although not profound, indicate interest and concern.)*

The physician who has many patients and little time is tortured by patients who are diffuse and vague. To manage this problem, physicians develop habits of asking leading questions, asking questions that include prompted answers (including multiple-choice lists) or questions that invite yes/no answers.

THERAPIST 1: Did you leave school because you had to work to help the family? *(A better approach is "I'd like to know about your decision to quit school.")*
THERAPIST 2: Did your mother think it was a good idea for you to quit school, or did she object? *(A better question is "What did your mother say about your decision to quit school?")*
THERAPIST 3: How much do you drink? A little wine with meals? *(A better question is "What is your usual use of alcohol?")*

The open-ended question has the greatest potential for eliciting information. Prompts and suggestions are appropriate when the patient is unable to respond to a broad question. Prompts that elicit a "no" answer or multiple-choice lists that fail to include a correct alternative may cause the patient to infer that the therapist does not understand.

The beginner therapist who has overcome the habit of asking questions is at risk of falling into unproductive agreeableness, always responding to the patient's most recent words. The therapist asks a question, the patient gives a partial answer and then moves to another topic, the therapist asks a question about that, and the process is repeated, with the therapist never having the opportunity to deal with anything useful. Beginning therapists are often easily put off because if a patient's answer is not adequate, they go on to another question instead of pursuing an answer to the initial question. In short, asking too many questions is not good form, but if a question is asked, it should not be abandoned without an attempt to get an answer. The therapist who does not attempt to understand the whole story sends the message that he or she does not really care. Compare the following two interactions:

THERAPIST 1: Do you have any thoughts about any issues or events that may have led up to your depression last year?
PATIENT 1: Nothing. It just happened. It came out of the blue.

THERAPIST 1: Have you ever felt suicidal? *(The therapist, if curious about what led to the depression, should have attempted to persist with that topic even though suicide is also an important issue.)*

THERAPIST 2: What was happening in your life in the month or so before the depression began? *(persisting with a general question that does not call on the patient to make cause-and-effect connections)*

PATIENT 2: Nothing special. I went to work. I came home. My husband was working. The kids were in school *(uninformative)*.

THERAPIST 2: Let's take them one at a time. What about work? What were you doing? What about coworkers? Any problems? Did anyone you care about leave? Was your assignment changed? Your supervisor? Advancement? *(By deliberately offering multiple-choice options, the therapist hints at topics that might be important.)*

PATIENT 2: Not really. Everything was routine *(uninformative)*.

THERAPIST 2: OK. Tell me about your husband and children at that time. What was going on? We are looking for things that might have been disturbing but that you might have brushed aside at the time without paying much attention. *(The prodding question is asked in a supportive way. Although suggesting answers to questions was described earlier as bad form, it may be used as a tactic for educating the patient about important issues and maintaining focus.)*

Seeking more complete information about what the patient is saying is a demonstration of interest and attention, so it is a supportive act, provided that the pursuit of additional information does not take on the quality of an attack. Emotionally attuned listening and clarification seeking can be very reassuring to a patient, and much more information may come forward in the interaction between the therapist and patient. The key to obtaining complete information is often the wonderful phrase "Give me an example."

PATIENT 1: If I get mad at work, I just don't go back.

THERAPIST 1: Give me an example. What was the incident that got to you?

PATIENT 1: It was nothing. I was working a counter. A customer was arguing with me.

THERAPIST 1: So a customer started to argue with you. Let's try to look at what happened. What did the customer say, and what did you say?

PATIENT 2: I have to do everything. My husband is helpless in the house. I come home from work and I have to get dinner, even though he's been home.

THERAPIST 2: What do you mean by "helpless?" Does he do any tasks at all?

PATIENT 3: No, I never get angry. I can't remember ever losing my temper.

THERAPIST 3: Can you describe some instance in which something displeased you a little?

Maintaining and Improving Self-Esteem

Maintaining or improving self-esteem is a major concern of supportive psychotherapy. One person helps the self-esteem of another person by conveying acceptance, approval, interest, respect, or admiration. The person whose daily life and relationships are lacking or deficient in these qualities may respond to any indication of their presence. The patient who cannot form relationships with others, who is avoided by others, or who perceives (perhaps correctly) that people look at him or her disapprovingly, finds in the therapist a person who is accepting and interested. The therapist's acceptance and respect are unspoken. The therapist communicates interest in the patient by making it evident that he or she remembers their conversations; recalls what the patient has said; and is aware of the patient's likes, dislikes, and attitudes. Acceptance is communicated by avoidance of arguing, denigrating, and criticizing—verbal interactions common to many relationships, including, unfortunately, many contacts between patients and health care providers.

Below are therapist responses that are negatively stated followed by responses that are more positive, congenial, and encouraging.

THERAPIST 1: It doesn't make any sense to get an MRI [magnetic resonance imaging] just because you forget people's names *(argument)*.
THERAPIST 2: Forgetting names is usually the first memory issue that healthy people experience. If that is the only problem, it's not caused by the sort of thing that shows up on an MRI *(respectful, reassuring)*.

THERAPIST 1: What are you trying to say? *(denigration)*
THERAPIST 2: OK, I am not sure I understand. Can you say more? *(encouraging clarification)*

THERAPIST 1: Didn't they tell you to take your medication every day? *(criticism)*
THERAPIST 2: A lot of the effect is lost if you don't take your medication every day. If the dosage is too large, we should discuss it. A smaller dosage might be the answer *(informative, nonjudgmental, inviting response)*.

In their efforts to boost or avoid lowering the patient's self-esteem, therapists need to avoid language that is overpowering (directly or by implication) and behavior that may make the patient feel diminished or helpless, such as pomposity, overelaborate speech, or ostentatiousness. The following are some overpowering statements:

THERAPIST 1: I'm trying to get you to understand….
THERAPIST 2: I'm going to medicate you.
THERAPIST 3: It's your imagination.

Here are better ways to express the same ideas:

THERAPIST 1: I hope I'm being clear.
THERAPIST 2: Let's talk about medication.
THERAPIST 3: When you hear something that people around you don't hear, it's not imagination; it's an event in your brain that's not triggered by something in the environment.

Questions that begin with the words *why* or *why didn't you* are often experienced as attacks, and they should be avoided (Pinsker 1997). In the course of growing up, most people learn that "Why did you do it?" is not so much a search for information as a rebuke for having committed a certain act. Similarly, "Why didn't you do it?" means "You should have done it." Attack is inimical to self-esteem. Alternatives to *why* questions might include the following:

THERAPIST 1: Can you explain how it was that you did it that way?
THERAPIST 2: When you dropped out of school, what was the reason?
THERAPIST 3: Was there something about your behavior that made them think it was necessary to call the police?

Attacking questions are accepted as a matter of course in most relationships, and they are certainly customary in conventional medical practice, so reasonable use of them will not destroy the therapy. The objective is to conduct therapy with finesse, thus enhancing the prospects for success. When possible, it is better to ask a general question than a narrow question. For example, "What is your usual use of alcohol?" is a better question than "Do you drink wine with meals?" It is also better practice, when possible, to ask questions in a way that elicits a positive response rather than a negative response. The therapist should not be a person to whom the patient must too often answer "No." Asking questions that are likely to be answered with a "no" implies that the therapist does not understand the patient.

The doctor-patient relationship involves a person who has the power to give help and a person who needs help. The doctor should give help in a skillful manner that minimizes the inherent inequality of the transaction and communicates respect for the patient. Respect is good for self-esteem and good for the therapeutic alliance. Giving the patient vague, dismissive explanations conveys lack of respect.

PATIENT 1: I think this medication is making me sleepy.
PHYSICIAN 1: It hasn't been a problem for most people. How's your appetite? *(dismissive)*

PATIENT 2: I don't feel any better.
PHYSICIAN 2: Well, you look better. *(If coupled with an explanation that depressed people look better before they feel better, this would be fine. As an abrupt response, it is dismissive and argumentative.)*

Even educated, sophisticated patients tend to tolerate disrespectful attitudes and behavior from health care providers because patients are dependent on health care providers and cannot risk animosity. The patient may employ the defenses of rationalization or denial in order to avoid awareness of resentment. For many individuals, the reality of needing care has a negative effect on self-esteem. The health care provider should not rub salt into the wound.

We recommend that therapists discuss with the patient the reasons for asking specific questions, explain to the patient the direction being taken, and ask the patient for agreement on topics to be discussed. We refer to these tactics as *setting the agenda* or *showing the map*. For patients, these tactics help to prevent both the anxiety that may be associated with going in unknown directions and the interrogatory atmosphere that reinforces the idea that the patient is in an inferior position.

Defenses

In the supportive approach, defenses are encouraged (supported) when they serve their unconscious purpose—protecting the individual from anxiety or other unpleasant affect. When therapy is primarily expressive, defenses are identified and examined to discover the underlying conflicts that made the defenses necessary. In supportive psychotherapy, defenses are questioned only when they are maladaptive. For example, a patient's denial as a strategy for not thinking about the inevitably fatal outcome of his or her own life is adaptive, whereas a patient's denial that leads to his or her refusal of potentially safe and beneficial treatment is maladaptive. In expressive psychotherapy, passive-aggressive behavior might be explored as an indicator of unconscious hostility and a need to control others; in supportive psychotherapy, the same behavior might be accepted as adaptive. When dealing with defenses, the situation is fluid—a therapist may support one defense and question another. Also, a therapist might recognize and not question a defense early in treatment but question it later in treatment.

In maintaining the supportive stance in the therapist-patient relationship, the therapist should consider it permissible and desirable to explore the meaning of the patient's actions and thoughts. Whether the therapist supports, ignores, or questions a statement that appears to reflect a defensive position depends on the current situation, including the context of the patient-therapist conversation (e.g., the therapist must consider whether to interrupt the patient to raise a question or to go along with the patient's flow). The following are examples of different responses:

> PATIENT: I hated being in the hospital. Every day someone would be acting up, and they'd jump on him with a needle. I was glad I wasn't that bad off.
> THERAPIST 1: Yeah *(accepts the defense without comment)*.
> THERAPIST 2: Maybe you were afraid on some level that it could happen to you. A lot of people equate mental illness with being out of control, so if they find themselves in a hospital because they have a mental illness, they are afraid they may be in danger of being out of control *(proposes an explanation for the defense, using the technique of normalization to lessen the impact)*.
> THERAPIST 3: Yes. Your condition was quite different. Severe depression is one thing; a psychotic episode is another. That wouldn't happen to you *(encourages the defense)*.

When does the therapist need to be expressive? Expressive techniques can be used without altering the supportive stance whenever the basic supportive techniques do not appear to be enough to accomplish the patient's goals and it appears that the patient's life can be improved by use of expressive techniques. As stated in Chapter 1, "Evolution of the Concept of Supportive Psychotherapy," the therapist must know whether his or her basic stance with a patient is supportive or expressive—the therapist cannot maintain both transference-encouraging neutrality and a real relationship at the same time.

Psychodynamic Assumptions

Many physicians begin psychiatric training without having had exposure to psychodynamics or any form of psychotherapy. Some trainees are from countries where psychodynamic thinking has not been widely disseminated. Trainees may not know what to talk about with a patient after completing the history, hoping that improvement will occur, in some way, if the patient talks about his or her past and feelings. For the absolute beginner (and no one else), we offer the following words about psychodynamics.

Psychodynamics is the interaction between conscious and unconscious elements of mental life. It is an explanation of the meaning of behavior. One of the tasks of psychotherapy is to create order out of symptoms and dysfunctions. To accomplish this task, the patient and therapist join in developing a history or narrative in which these symptoms and dysfunctions make sense. Cause-and-effect connections are established. Different schools of psychodynamic thinking may derive different explanations at times. The process of making a comprehensible story may be what matters most.

The following are a few examples of psychodynamic formulations.

Case Illustration 1

David, a man who is ordinarily self-sufficient and cheerful, becomes demanding and uncooperative when hospitalized following a heart attack, although he has been reassured that his prognosis is very good. A psychodynamic hypothesis might be that the passive, somewhat helpless role of hospital patient is anxiety provoking, and David is attempting to compensate by assuming an overbearing attitude. Because he is unaware that the enforced passivity is behind his unusual behavior, his behavior is considered to be unconscious.

Case Illustration 2

After being criticized by his parents for watching television all night, Mark, a patient with schizophrenia, becomes angry with his parents and stops taking his antipsychotic medication. According to his chart, he has been educated about taking the medication and has verbalized understanding. He is not aware that "forgetting" to take his medication may be psychologically motivated defiance.

Case Illustration 3

After returning home for Thanksgiving during his first year of college, Zach, a healthy teenager, provokes a big argument the day before he leaves, with the consequence that he is angry when he leaves. He is not aware that part (not all) of him would like to stay home and be dependent. By going away angry, he is protected from the sadness that is part of his departure.

Case Illustration 4

Susan comes irregularly for clinic visits, each time giving a detailed account of how other people mistreat her. After many attempts to get Susan to examine her role in causing or maintaining at least some of her troubles, the therapist raises the question of why Susan has sought psychotherapy and whether it should be discontinued. A psychodynamic hypothesis might be that because repeating familiar patterns is an anxiety-reducing element of human behavior, Susan may be setting up a situation in which she will be rejected, thus confirming her expectations about relationships with people.

Unrecognized Emotions

An assumption of psychodynamically oriented therapies is that unrecognized emotions are often responsible for current unpleasant feelings or maladaptive behavior. At times, simply becoming aware of the emotions may provide relief. More often, the discovery of the feeling must be followed by conscious decisions about more effective methods of coping—this is the adaptive skills focus of supportive psychotherapy. In the past, many patients' symptoms were related to what they perceived as unacceptable sexual feelings—a problem that is less common today. Unrecognized anger is a frequently seen problem ("getting the anger out" was once proposed as a simple, curative tactic but is now recognized as counterproductive). Other often-hidden feelings might be grief that was not experienced at the time of an important loss, guilt or hopelessness, or a wish to be admired or to be obeyed. Some individuals are scarcely aware of any feelings at all; the term *alexithymia* has been used to describe these patients. For patients with alexithymia, an important objective is to recognize, acknowledge, identify, and label emotions (Misch 2000). The general task is to incorporate awareness of feelings into the fabric of memories and current life.

The beginner therapist often asks, "How did it feel?" or "How does it feel?" in response to almost anything the patient says, with no intent or plan about what to do with the answer. If the therapist and patient are working on the problem of unrecognized feelings, the patient's feelings connected to events in the past should be explored. Feelings should be explored if the therapist and patient are examining coping strategies or if the therapist is seeking opportunities to expand his or her empathic understanding. Often, with respect to a current feeling, the question to discuss must be "What is going to be done about it?" The question "What did you think?" is as useful as "What did you feel?" because it pertains to thought process, reality testing, or adaptive skills.

In short, a person who knows thoughts but does not know feelings needs to feel more, whereas a person who feels too much needs to think and evaluate more. Therapeutic dialogue often involves both feelings and thoughts; jumping to adaptive solutions without understanding the patient's emotional response is just as wrong as ignoring adaptive solutions altogether. However, supportive psychotherapy often focuses on thoughts, especially for more impaired patients who have problems with feelings and require a more cognitive focus.

The question "How did you feel?" is pertinent when it initiates discussion of how the patient dealt with the feeling or, if there was no feeling, discussion of the possibility that this lack of feeling is of itself an important finding.

> PATIENT: I asked the guy next door to go to the mall with me, but he said he didn't have time. He doesn't have any more to do than I do.
> THERAPIST: How did you feel about that?
> PATIENT: It's all right. He doesn't have to. *(evasive, denying emotional response)*
> THERAPIST: You're right. He doesn't have to. That's a correct analysis *(praise)*. But you're offering an analysis when I asked about your feelings *(confrontation; implied question)*.

PATIENT: I didn't feel anything.

THERAPIST: You describe a situation in which most people would feel disappointment or anger. That reaction won't control the other person, but it's important to know what your feelings are because
when you don't, you can't make good decisions about things that
affect you *(teaching, normalizing)*.

Maladaptive Behaviors

Another tenet of psychodynamically oriented therapy is that people often
follow patterns of behavior that were appropriate when established but
now have become maladaptive. For example, during adolescence, when
it is important to reduce emotional dependency on parents, many people
assume a belligerent or defiant style. This attitude may be appropriate at
age 16 but may become a continual source of trouble if it persists at age 26,
46, or 66. Some people, once they see that they are clinging to a pattern
of behavior that is familiar and understandable but no longer useful, are
able, with determined effort, to change their habitual responses. Cognitive-behavioral therapy focuses on the assumptions associated with patterns of thought and provides tactics for overcoming these assumptions.
Although cognitive and psychodynamic approaches are usually taught separately, tactics of both approaches are integrated in everyday treatment.

The search for patterns that may explain symptoms or maladaptive behavior is the expressive component of supportive-expressive psychotherapy. Once the therapist has elicited the history, he or she is concerned first
about feelings and assumptions that are present but unexpressed, then
about feelings and assumptions that are lightly concealed, and later about
feelings and assumptions that have been truly hidden. A long-familiar
analogy is that psychotherapy is like peeling an onion.

Psychogenetics and Early Life Experiences

Psychodynamic explanations tell about the interplay of factors in current
life; they do not explain the origins of the forces, emotions, or assumptions
that affect behavior. *Psychogenetics* is the search for these origins. When a
therapist says that a man who seeks to have as many sexual relationships as
possible is hypersexual, the therapist is offering a diagnostic impression
(not a DSM diagnosis). When the therapist says that the patient acts this
way to compensate for insecurity about his masculinity, the therapist is
making a psychodynamic hypothesis. When the therapist says that the patient is insecure because he was afraid of his overbearing father, the therapist is proposing a genetic hypothesis. If the patient is readily able to form
relationships but always ends them by discovering faults in his partner and

shifting from loving behavior to quarreling, a psychodynamic possibility is that he is unconsciously fearful of closeness or intimacy.

The interpersonal and emotional experiences of early life are important in the development of the individual and his or her problems. Creating a meaningful autobiography is in itself useful because during the process, what may have appeared to be random events become connected into a meaningful story.

The problem for the beginning therapist is that some patients talk endlessly about their terrible childhoods, emphasizing how they suffered various forms of maltreatment. The inexperienced therapist may feel hopeful that some good will come from allowing ongoing talk by a patient who is avoiding any discussion about changing his or her patterns or manner of relating to people. Venting can be a legitimate supportive tactic that is useful when the patient has been unable to put painful experiences into words, perhaps because he or she has been afraid to do so or because no one has been available to listen and understand. Recounting the same story also may be adaptive when the patient's goal is limited to relapse prevention and the therapist's objective is to preserve the status quo; however, such retelling is maladaptive when the goal is to improve the patient's life. Retelling can be especially maladaptive in individuals with a significant trauma history for whom the retelling is accompanied by tremendous distress.

Mode of Action

Attempts to achieve the supportive psychotherapy objectives of improved ego function and adaptive skills involve teaching, encouragement, exhortation, modeling, and anticipatory guidance. People in general, not only patients, respond to teaching and instruction if they want to learn, if they want to improve their lot, and if they trust the teacher. People may cooperate with the teacher to please him or her. Such cooperation has been described in psychoanalytic writing as a *transference cure*. The Menninger psychotherapy research project found that changes that appeared to come about for this reason proved stable and durable (Wallerstein 1989). Sometimes, advice or instruction from another person, especially an authority figure, is a catalyst, allowing the patient to accomplish change that he or she had already formulated.

The many approaches to psychotherapy have produced competing claims. Extensive research has aimed to discover the active ingredient in psychotherapy. Because all therapies have been found to be effective, an important research question emerged: "What do all therapies have in common?" A number of common factors have been found, of which the therapeutic relationship or therapeutic alliance is perhaps the most important (de Jonghe et al. 1992; Frank and Frank 1991; Rosenzweig 1936; Westerman et al. 1995). If there is a good alliance between patient and therapist, therapy is helpful. If there is not a good alliance, little is accomplished. Therefore, the therapist must make deliberate efforts to encourage a good relationship and avoid actions that are inimical to a good relationship (for further discussion, see Chapter 6). The patient's experience of "an atmosphere of warmth, hope, caring, and authenticity" is important in the therapeutic interaction (Brenner 2012, p. 262).

The patient's transference may cause him or her to unconsciously perceive the therapist as having attributes associated with unpleasant interactions in the past. The therapist, however, does not respond as the figure from the past did, and in time, the old feelings become muted, and the patient no longer needs to replay new relationships according to the old emotional script. According to theory, this result is accomplished without explicit analysis. Alexander and French (1946) introduced the term *corrective emotional experience* to describe this process. Corrective emotional experiences may occur at any point on the spectrum of psychopathology and the spectrum of psychotherapies. Gabbard (2017) summarized current thinking: "Now most clinicians and researchers feel that insight through interpretation has historically been idealized and that change also occurs through the experience of a new kind of relationship in psychotherapy" (p. 94).

Education and instruction are potent agents for bringing about change in people's lives. Advice and instruction are most likely to be followed when given by a person whom the individual trusts and respects. The skillful therapist or teacher gives instruction that is needed at the time when it can be absorbed and used. The patient's mother may have said, "Clean your room." The psychotherapist teaches, "It's not good for your self-esteem for you to be surrounded by evidence that you can't keep some order in your life." Sometimes, this approach is all that is required to bring about change.

In the 1960s, learning theory, which previously had been of more interest to science-minded psychologists than to clinical psychiatrists, was presented as the theoretical basis of behavior therapy (an approach that had been demonstrated to be effective for many disorders), contrary to predictions based on theories underlying psychoanalytic therapy. Change, initiated by a therapy based on an educational approach, was found to occur even if neither patient nor therapist understood the historical origins of the problem. Education and instruction have been accepted throughout history as strategies for changing behavior and thought, although such changes cannot be guaranteed or predicted—when a patient mentions a former therapist, it is remarkable how often the patient tells us what that therapist told him or her to do. Research on the process of learning, although focused on formal education, has led to observations that new information is linked to what is already known, that retrieving information repeatedly enhances subsequent recall, and that elaborating on the material contributes to learning (deWinstanley and Bjork 2002). Although the field of learning theory has contributed potentially useful ways of explaining the process of education and change, such as critical reflection (Mezirow 1998), these ideas have not percolated through psychotherapy education.

The techniques of cognitive and behavior therapies are used somewhat informally in supportive psychotherapy, usually without the emphasis on homework. Faulty cognition and the persistence of automatic thoughts are recognized as processes that often contribute to symptom formation and to maladaptive behavior. In supportive psychotherapy, the therapist may address faulty cognition when the patient is able to accept the self-scrutiny entailed. Desensitization, a central theme of behavior therapy, may contribute to the beneficial effect of history-oriented psychotherapy in that it involves repeated safe exposure to once painful memories (Goldberg and Green 1986).

Patients at the most supportive end of the supportive-expressive continuum find that simply being able to talk to a person who is interested and accepting minimizes the loneliness in their lives. Being able to talk about experiences and worries brings relief, even when the patients receive no reassuring or normalizing response. Identification with the therapist as a reasonable, stable individual may promote stability and better relationships with others. When associated with events that have been concealed, venting can be curative. Repeating the same story month after month may be comforting for the patient, even when he or she makes no progress. From the medical perspective, maintaining the status quo may be a reasonable and responsible objective. At the same time, however, the therapist hopes to find opportunities to help the patient improve his or her situation.

The concept of *change* appears throughout the literature on psychotherapy. At one end of the spectrum, change means lasting personality change. At the other end, desirable changes may involve changing specific behaviors, such as sitting in front of the television all day, skipping medications, spending money foolishly, remaining in a bad environment, or failing to control children. If simple advice is all that is needed to get the patient to change habitual behavior, it is not necessary to examine possible causes of the behavior. Often, however, there are obstacles to bringing about change that the patient does not verbalize. If the therapist is to give useful advice, he or she must be familiar with the psychological and emotional problems that may be operating.

> THERAPIST 1: The last time you were here, we talked about the support group, and you said you were going to talk to the social worker about it. I wonder what happened that you didn't. (*"What happened?" is not as attacking as "Why?"*)
> PATIENT 1: I don't know. I had trouble with my car. I had to go to the dentist.
> THERAPIST 1: I know a lot of people have trouble doing too many things in one week. It's also an easy habit to get into and not a good one (*normalizing, exhorting, judgmental*).
>
> THERAPIST 2: People who have not been able to do much for a long time—it can happen with illness—become fearful of doing new things. They think that they will do something wrong or won't know how to fit in. Does that make any sense? (*teaching; confronting—i.e., bringing to the patient's attention feelings or thoughts that had been outside his or her awareness*)
> PATIENT 2: I get very nervous when I meet new people.
> THERAPIST 2: So we need to find a way to deal with the nervousness that will make it possible for you to have the interview with the social worker. Then you can determine whether the group might be of use to you (*scolding replaced by acceptance; moving toward constructive efforts*).

These dialogues illustrate how even in work with the most impaired individuals, the therapist must explore feelings and ideas of which the patient has not been aware. This exploration is an expressive element. If the therapy is to go beyond the simplest take-it-or-leave-it advice and beyond criticizing the patient for being noncompliant, the therapy must take into account psychodynamic considerations.

Films and plays of the 1950s often show a patient in psychotherapy or psychoanalysis discovering an early traumatic experience, after which recovery is immediate. In real life, once such discoveries are made, a patient typically must work hard to change his or her ways of thinking and responding. Although the importance of explaining origins is not as great as once thought, an explanation of origins still has its uses. For the patient to own a meaningful personal story is to give him or her a feeling of mastery, and the creation of the story is a shared task for patient and therapist. From the scientific point of view, the therapist can never be certain whether the patient's story agrees with what actually happened—or whether the apparent cause-and-effect connections are valid. As an example of the latter, people who have been emotionally and physically abused when they were children are more likely to be abusive adults than are those who never received such treatment—but this result is not inevitable. Therapists, as well as the general public, often blur the distinction between anecdote and group data. The methods of cognitive-behavioral therapy, many of which have been incorporated into supportive psychotherapy, may be the principal approach once the patient sees that the behavior that is causing distress is the outcome of a plausible story. Misch (2000) advises the supportive therapist to be like a good parent. The supportive therapist is advised to comfort, soothe, encourage, and nurture the patient; to set limits; and to confront self-destructive behaviors, all while encouraging the patient's growth and self-sufficiency.

Conclusion

Supportive psychotherapy is conducted in conversational style, involving examination of the patient's current and past experiences, responses, and feelings. In supportive psychotherapy, the therapist is active and inquires and responds in ways that seek to bolster the patient's strengths. Although the initial focus is on self-esteem, ego function, and adaptive skills, as with other forms of psychotherapy, the therapeutic alliance may be the most important element. The therapist seeks to expand the patient's self-mastery by helping him or her to become aware of thoughts and feelings that had been outside awareness and to provide specific suggestions for more adaptive living.

Assessment, Case Formulation, and Goal Setting

3

Assessment

The process of evaluation and case formulation is essential for all psychotherapeutic approaches. The most important objective of the evaluation process is to establish a positive therapeutic relationship (alliance) with the patient. The patient is more likely to see himself or herself as a partner in the diagnostic endeavor when the therapeutic relationship is positive, which will lead to a more thorough and informative evaluation. A positive therapeutic relationship can also further the patient's interest in and commitment to psychotherapy.

As the patient evaluation unfolds, the evaluator can establish a positive relationship with the patient by displaying an interest in what the patient is saying. This is accomplished by listening attentively and providing feedback on symptoms, problems, conflicts, and relationships. The evaluator should respond to the patient with empathy, interest, and responsive and explanatory comments so that the patient can begin to understand his or her problems and conflicts.

A central objective of the assessment process is to diagnose the patient's illness and describe the patient's problems so that the individual can be treated appropriately. A thorough evaluation should help the clinician select the appropriate treatment approach. The treatment plan should be individualized to meet the needs and goals of the patient.

The supportive-expressive continuum, introduced in Chapter 1, "Evolution of the Concept of Supportive Psychotherapy," is a useful way of thinking about and conceptualizing the evaluation process. In this chapter, we combine the psychotherapy continuum (lower labels on Figure 3–1) with an impairment or psychopathology continuum (upper labels on Figure 3–1). Supportive psychotherapy is indicated for patients on the left side of the continuum (higher levels of psychopathology), whereas expressive psychotherapy is better suited for patients on the right side of the continuum (healthier patients).

When a therapist meets a patient for the first time, the therapist generally does not know the extent of the patient's impairment, psychopathology, or strengths. Therefore, the therapist should begin the initial interview by attempting to understand why the patient has come for treatment. The therapist should thoroughly evaluate the current problems and past history of each patient. The technical approach will vary, from the use of a more supportive approach for patients with higher levels of psychopathology to a more expressive approach for healthier patients. If, in the course of working with a patient, the therapist finds that the patient has more significant psychopathology, the therapist may have to quickly move into a more supportive mode. The degree of disturbance encountered during the initial interview will determine how the clinician proceeds in that interview.

In this conceptualization, supportive psychotherapy is indicated for patients with high levels of psychopathology, whereas expressive psychotherapy is better suited for healthier patients. We have found in our clinical and research work that supportive and expressive psychotherapies produce similar results in patients across the psychopathology continuum (see Chapter 9, "Evaluating Competence and Outcome Research"). Therefore, supportive psychotherapy is indicated for a wide variety of disorders across the psychopathology continuum (for a full discussion of inclusion and exclusion criteria for supportive psychotherapy, see Chapter 5, "General Framework of Supportive Psychotherapy"). The efficacy of supportive psychotherapy in higher-functioning patients is especially enhanced when expressive and cognitive-behavioral techniques are integrated into a supportive approach (Winston and Winston 2002).

The patient evaluation should be comprehensive and, if possible, should be completed during an extended first session of at least 60 minutes. At the end of the evaluation, the therapist should understand the patient's problems, interpersonal relationships, everyday functioning, and psychological structure. The evaluation interview should not be a series of

Level of impairment

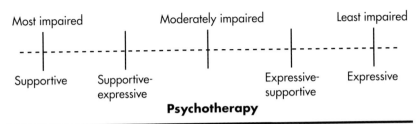

Figure 3–1. Impairment-psychotherapy continuum.

questions and answers. Instead, it should be more of an exploration of the patient's life. The interview should be therapeutic, to help motivate the patient for treatment and promote the therapeutic alliance. In a supportive approach, a therapist may make an evaluation therapeutic by using appropriate interventions, such as empathic clarifications and confrontations.

The evaluation should begin with an exploration of the patient's presenting problems or areas of disturbance. Presenting problems may include symptoms, relationship and self difficulties, work or school issues, medical problems, and substance abuse issues. Generally, symptoms should be explored first so that the clinician is informed about the extent of the patient's psychopathology. Exploring symptoms first is also helpful to the patient because symptoms are what patients care about. Information about symptoms will enable the clinician to adjust the evaluation interview to the patient's level of psychopathology. With some patients, the extent of psychopathology will be clear from the start, particularly if the patient has a loss of reality testing. With other patients, psychopathology may be less discernible and more time may be required.

After the presenting problems have been clearly delineated, the therapist should explore the patient's history. We want to emphasize that therapists should not move on to an exploration of the patient's history until all of his or her current problems and symptoms have been thoroughly explored. Patients will often bring up an important experience from their past while discussing a current problem. When this occurs, the evaluator should say, "What you are bringing up is important and I want to hear about it, but let's first finish exploring the current issues in your life."

Exploration of the patient's history can be accomplished in many ways but should be systematic and should cover relationships with parents, other caretakers, siblings, grandparents, and other people in the patient's life and household. Descriptions of these individuals should also be obtained. Important issues to inquire about include trauma; separation and loss; medical problems, psychiatric illness, and substance abuse (in the patient and first-degree relatives); geographic moves; family belief systems; school history; sexual development and experiences; identity issues; and financial matters. Past psychiatric treatment, including psychotherapy and pharmacotherapy, should be explored, as should the patient's response to the therapist, because this knowledge can alert the therapist to potential problems in the therapeutic alliance.

As soon as the therapist determines that the patient should be treated with supportive or supportive-expressive psychotherapy, the evaluation interview should promote the objectives of supportive psychotherapy. These objectives are to ameliorate symptoms and to maintain, restore, or improve self-esteem, adaptive skills, and ego or psychological functions (Pinsker et al. 1991).

A useful method of conceptualizing dynamic psychotherapy, which encompasses both supportive and expressive approaches, involves the triangles of conflict and person. The focus of the triangle of conflict (Freud 1926/1959; Malan 1979) (Figure 3–2) is on wishes, needs, and feelings that are warded off by defenses and anxiety. In this model, a therapist who is pursuing a patient's feeling is at the wish/need/feeling point of the triangle. As is often the case, the patient may respond defensively to the exploration of feeling (second point of the triangle). The patient also may respond with anxiety (the third point of the triangle) because of fear of the conflicted feeling.

In the triangle of person (Malan 1979; Menninger 1958) (Figure 3–3), the three points all relate to people and include individuals in the patient's current life and past life and the therapist or transference figure. In expressive or exploratory psychotherapy, the therapist tends to work on conflict situations using the triangles to explore wishes, needs, and feelings that the patient may have in relation to an important person in his or her life. When defenses interfere with exploration, the therapist addresses them. Present and past issues are addressed, and the transference relationship and its exploration are emphasized.

In supportive psychotherapy, the triangles of conflict and person are used differently. In the triangle of conflict, feelings generally are not pursued, anxiety is diminished, and defenses are strengthened. In the triangle of person, the real relationship with the therapist is emphasized, and the therapist works primarily on present persons and current issues in the patient's life.

The following video vignette, which is presented as an enactment and is available online at www.appi.org/Winston, illustrates the use of supportive therapy in an initial evaluation (see Video Vignette 1).

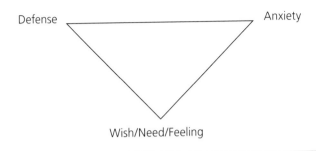

Figure 3–2.   Triangle of conflict.

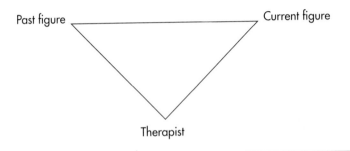

Figure 3–3.   Triangle of person.

 Video Vignette 1: Assessment

Mary, a 42-year-old woman, was referred by her primary care physician because of depression, beginning at age 24, and a number of other problems. She recently went through a divorce and is having a great deal of difficulty finding a job. She has a history of multiple episodes of depression and was hospitalized once for suicidal depression.

THERAPIST: So as you know, Dr. Perry sent you to see me for an evaluation. Can you tell me what the problem is?

MARY: I just don't feel right. I don't know. I can't seem to get anything done *(responds in a vague manner that could be defensive or a sign of disorganization)*.

THERAPIST: So you don't feel right and you haven't been able to get anything done and you're at a loss *(responds with a supportive clarification that helps Mary to focus on the question at hand)*.

MARY: Yeah, I just sit around. I can't get started. Everything is just a mess. I feel so bad [*becomes tearful*].

The therapist recognizes that Mary may be depressed and asks a series of questions to determine whether this is so and, if so, the extent of the depression.

- Have you been feeling down? Have you been crying or feeling tearful?
- What is your energy level like? Have you been tired a lot?
- Are you anxious, fearful, jumpy?
- What about your sleep patterns? Are you having problems falling asleep or are you sleeping too much?
- How is your appetite? Are you losing or gaining weight?
- Are you maintaining your social relationships? Do you find pleasure in your life? Do you go out? Are you working or having difficulty at work?
- What is your attitude about the future? Do you feel hopeful?
- Have you wished you were dead or wished you could go to sleep and not wake up? Have you had any thoughts of killing yourself?
- Have you been thinking about how you might do this? Have you had these thoughts and had some intention of acting on them (Posner et al. 2009)?
- Are you able to have sexual relations? Is sex pleasurable?

Mary responds that for the past 2 months, she has been consistently downhearted, tearful, fatigued, and pessimistic about the future and has had difficulty concentrating. She has trouble falling asleep, consistently awakens during early morning hours, and is unable to get back to sleep. Her appetite is poor, and she has lost approximately 10 pounds in the past 2 weeks. She is preoccupied with death and has thoughts of killing herself but has no defined plan. She rarely goes out, nothing gives her pleasure or satisfaction, and she has no sexual desire or interest. She stopped working a few weeks ago. She has never had a manic or hypomanic episode. In the past, she was treated with antidepressants, and during her last episode, she was treated with paroxetine. Mary stopped taking her medication 6 months ago.

The therapist recognizes that Mary is in the midst of a major depressive episode and has some cognitive difficulties. This level of psychopathology places Mary on the left side of the continuum (see Figure 3–1), which indicates that the therapist should continue the evaluation in a supportive mode.

THERAPIST: So it sounds to me as if you've been feeling depressed. From what you've told me, it seems you're depressed now and have been depressed several times in the past. These things you're describing—tearfulness, fatigue, difficulty concentrating, trouble sleeping, feeling bad, having a hard time getting started—all these things are symptoms of depression. *(**Naming the problem makes it understandable and reassures the patient that each symptom is not a separate condition.**)*

MARY: I just feel so hopeless and horrible. I feel like nothing's ever going to get better. It's just that there are so many things...so many things that are bothering me. *(**The therapist has begun to educate Mary about her depression. Education is important in all forms of psychotherapy, especially in supportive treatment. Education provides the patient with knowledge about his or her difficulties and also demonstrates the therapist's interest and understanding, thereby promoting the therapeutic alliance.**)*

Next, the therapist explores how the current episode of depression began.

THERAPIST: We should try to look at this episode of depression. How long ago did it start? *(**proposed agenda**)*

MARY: Um, it got really bad 2 months ago, but I have to tell you I haven't been feeling good, probably for the past year. I don't feel myself.

THERAPIST: Did anything in particular happen? *(**continues to focus**)*

MARY [*tearful*]: My husband [Edward], who I've been married to for 14 years, I just found out that he had an affair with this woman that he works with, and he had the affair, and he left me. That's all I can say *(**begins to reveal important material that may have contributed to the onset of her depression**)*.

THERAPIST: I can see that this is really hard for you *(**empathic support**)*.

MARY: It's worse. I don't know what I did wrong. I feel so stupid. I feel I can't do anything. I can't go to work. I can't face the people. The people at work will think that I'm pathetic, and I'm too ashamed to tell anyone. I don't like to talk about it *(**indicates that her husband's infidelity and his leaving her led to a series of automatic [negative] thoughts**)*.

THERAPIST: So have you been able to continue at your job? *(**early focus on adaptive activity**)*

MARY: Well, it's been a struggle. It has been really hard.

THERAPIST: What do you think your coworkers might be thinking about you? *(**begins to explore Mary's automatic thoughts**)*

MARY: They think I'm pathetic.... I used to call my husband all the time from work. I felt so lonely and I felt scared that I couldn't do things right, and he would get so angry at me and he would say, "Why are you calling me? Why are you bothering me? Can't you do anything for yourself?"

THERAPIST: You've been feeling incompetent?

MARY: I feel so incompetent and...

THERAPIST: Can you give me a specific example of this? *(The therapist asks for a specific example because remaining at an abstract or general level promotes vagueness and loss of focus.)*

MARY: Oh, God… I mean, I was feeling incompetent. I remember this one time when I was at work and I fell and hit my head, and my head was bleeding and I needed stitches, and I called my husband to come help me and bring me to the doctor to get stitches, and he got angry at me and told me that he was busy and not to bother him and that I can't do anything right. I just felt so useless after that *(provides a clear interpersonal example)*.

THERAPIST: So you reached out to your husband for help and not only did he not help you, but he also put you down for it. This contributed to making you feel incompetent? *(summarizes patient's story)*

MARY: Well, yeah. I can't do anything right. I can't do anything right…yeah.

THERAPIST: I think that most people in that situation would ask for help and reach out to somebody. So I think that maybe you are making an erroneous judgment about yourself *(normalizing and then clarifying Mary's automatic thinking)*.

MARY: You think so?

THERAPIST: Perhaps this is a pattern with you? *(The therapist asks if this might be her habitual manner of behaving.)*

MARY: Maybe…I don't know?

The therapist has elicited a concrete example of an interaction with Mary's husband, an interaction that led her to think of herself as incompetent and helpless. This way of thinking is an example of automatic thoughts, which are quite common in depression. Mary's thought processes would constitute an important area on which to concentrate in supportive therapy for this type of disorder. In this instance, the therapist has attempted to point out that Mary's negative thinking was faulty, but the therapist has done so in a supportive manner by asking if Mary agreed. In subsequent sessions, the therapist should help Mary test her automatic thoughts herself.

The therapist then goes on to explore Mary's relationship with Edward, the history of their marriage, and her past history. Mary is in the throes of a major depressive disorder and has had four previous major depressive episodes as well as milder, chronic depression for most of her life. Serious difficulties in the interpersonal sphere, as well as personality problems, limit her ability to function. The therapist, a psychiatrist, concluded that Mary would benefit from medication and a supportive psychotherapy approach employing some cognitive-behavioral techniques. The therapist explained how both approaches—medication and psychotherapy—would be helpful in treating Mary's depression, anxiety, and problems in day-to-day functioning. Mary agreed with these immediate treatment goals and stated that she thinks the medication and psychotherapy are worth a try. The therapist explained when the medication will begin to work and have maximum effect and discussed possible side effects of the medication.

Diagnostic Evaluation

- Major depressive disorder, recurrent, moderate to severe
- Dependent personality disorder

Case Formulation

For each patient, the treatment approach should be based on the central issues emerging from the assessment and case formulation. The *case formulation* is an explanation of the patient's symptoms and psychosocial functioning. The therapist's formulation governs what interventions will be used as well as which issues in the patient-therapist dialogue will be selected for attention. Case formulation depends on an accurate and thorough assessment of the patient. Having a sense of the underlying issues at the start enhances the therapist's ability to respond empathically. At the same time, empathy for the patient helps the therapist guide and plan therapy effectively. The initial formulation is tentative and must be modified as more is learned about the patient during the course of psychotherapy.

Although the DSM-5 (American Psychiatric Association 2013a) diagnosis is an important element of the formulation, it is by no means the whole story. The diagnosis does not illuminate an individual's adaptive or maladaptive characteristics such as disappointments, his or her capacity for relationships, and how the individual thinks about and interprets life's events, nor does the diagnosis explain the unique life history of an individual. The DSM diagnosis alone does not fully explain the patient or the problem.

The following case formulation approaches are derived from psychoanalytic theory, including interpersonal and relational approaches, as well as cognitive-behavioral approaches. In the following subsections, we discuss the following case formulation approaches (Table 3–1): structural, genetic, dynamic, and cognitive-behavioral. Supportive psychotherapy uses elements of all these therapeutic approaches but differs in how these elements are used. For example, a patient's conflict may be clearly understood and formulated by the therapist but never or only partially explored in psychotherapy. Although these approaches have always been described

Table 3–1.   Types and foci of case formulations

Type	Focus
Structural	Concentrates on fixed aspects of an individual's personality within a functional context; assesses strengths and weaknesses and overall level of psychopathology
Genetic	Explores early development and life events that may explain the patient's current situation
Dynamic	Highlights the content of an individual's current conflicts and relates it to a primary lifelong or core conflict; examines mental and/or emotional tensions that may be conscious or unconscious
Cognitive-behavioral	Attends to the individual's automatic thoughts (based on the person's core beliefs or negative schemas) and how they can be addressed to change thoughts, behaviors, and moods

separately, a great deal of overlap exists, so some repetition occurs in the descriptions.

Structural Approach

A structural case formulation (Table 3–2) attempts to capture the relatively fixed characteristics of an individual's personality, which is understood within a functional context (in contrast with genetic and dynamic approaches, which are more content based). Assessment of an individual's strengths and weaknesses and overall level of psychopathology helps determine the clinician's technical approach. A thorough structural assessment enables the clinician to determine with some degree of accuracy where to place the patient on the impairment-psychotherapy continuum (see Figure 3–1).

Structural functions have been grouped together using Freud's (1923/1961) structural approach of id, ego, and superego. These agencies refer to the inner life of the patient. The following description of psychological or ego functions is based on the work of Beres (1956) and Bellak (1958). These categories are not mutually exclusive; there is a great deal of overlap.

Relation to Reality

Beres (1956) and Bellak (1958) described reality testing and sense of reality as major components of relation to reality. The term *reality testing* describes an individual's ability to assess reality. Reality testing is im-

---

Table 3–2. Components of the structural approach (ego and superego)

Ego functions

  Relation to reality

  Object relations

  Affects

  Impulse control

  Defenses

  Thought processes

  Autonomous functions (perception, intention, intelligence, language, and motor development)

  Synthetic function (ability to form a cohesive whole or gestalt)

Superego functions

  Conscience, morals, and ideals

---

paired in the presence of faulty judgment and is grossly disturbed in the presence of hallucinations or delusions. Sense of reality relates to a person's ability to distinguish self from other; presence of this ability indicates a stable and cohesive body image. Examples of disturbances in this function are depersonalization, derealization, and identity problems.

Disturbances in relation to reality indicate significant structural problems that place the patient on the left side of the impairment-psychotherapy continuum (see Figure 3–1). Such disturbances should point the clinician in the direction of a more supportive approach. Impaired relation to reality is a key indicator of structural deficits and should always be thoroughly explored.

Object Relations

Object relations refers to a person's capacity to relate in a meaningful way to significant individuals in his or her life. The function includes the ability to form intimate relationships, tolerate separation and loss, and maintain independence and autonomy. It also involves the sense of self and the ability to form a cohesive and stable self-image without diminishing or overidealizing self or other.

A patient's relationships with others form the foundation of the psychological functions constituting the structural approach. In all forms of psychotherapy, evaluation of object relations is central in determining a patient's placement on the impairment-psychotherapy continuum. Patients who are withdrawn and not interested in others or who have narcissistic, highly dependent, or chaotic relationships generally require a more supportive approach and therefore are on the left side of the continuum. Individuals who have had at least one meaningful give-and-take relationship tend to be on the right side of the continuum.

Affects, Impulse Control, and Defenses

Affects are complex psychophysiological states composed of subjective feelings and physiological accompaniments such as crying, blushing, sweating, posture, facial expression, and tone of voice. The range of affects includes excitement, joy, surprise, fear, anger, rage, irritation, anguish, shame, humiliation, sadness, and depression. The individual's ability to experience a wide range of affects at some depth and to differentiate between affects (as opposed to lumping them into a single feeling such as primitive rage) need to be assessed. Does the individual experience a wide variety and range of affects? Is the individual able to tolerate love, anger, joy, sadness, and humiliation? What are the predominant affects (Friedman and Lister 1987), and how regularly are they invoked?

The capacity to control impulses and to modulate affect in an adaptive manner indicates a well-functioning defensive structure. When impulse control is faulty, the individual may engage in socially unacceptable behavior, such as physically or verbally lashing out at others or making inappropriate demands. The ability to delay gratification and to tolerate frustration is another important aspect of impulse control.

Defenses mediate between a person's wishes, needs, and feelings and both internal prohibitions and the external world. Individuals tend to use the same kinds of behavior as patterned responses in reaction to perceived danger, difficult situations, or painful affects. Defenses are conceptualized as having both a developmental and a hierarchical organization. Three levels of defenses have been described: immature, intermediate, and mature. Examples of immature defenses are projection, hypochondriasis, acting out, sarcasm, and avoidance. Intermediate defenses include forgetting, intellectualization, displacement, and rationalization. Among the mature defenses are altruism, anticipation, suppression, sublimation, and humor (Vaillant 1977,). Primitive defenses, poor impulse control, severe affective instability, and shallow affect are indicators of structural deficits that place an individual on the left side of the continuum and suggest the need for a more supportive approach.

Thought Processes

The ability to think clearly, logically, and abstractly should be assessed. High levels of primary process or primitive thinking are a good indicator of severe psychopathology. Significant limitations in the ability to think logically suggest the need for a more supportive approach as opposed to an exploratory one. Dysfunctional and automatic thoughts should be identified so that cognitive-behavioral approaches can be applied.

Autonomous Functions

Autonomous functions—perception, intention, intelligence, language, and motor development—are believed to develop in a relatively conflict-free manner (Hartmann 1939/1958). Although these functions generally are not impaired in patients on the right side of the impairment-psychotherapy continuum, they can be affected in patients with significant psychopathology.

Synthetic Function

Synthetic function (Nunberg 1931) is the individual's ability to organize himself or herself and the world in a productive manner so that the individual can function in a harmonious and integrated way. Synthetic function is the psychological ability to form a cohesive whole, or gestalt, by putting together and organizing the other functions. For example, a young man meets several men and women for the first time at a dinner party. He engages each individual in a friendly and open manner with an appropriate affect. He is thoughtful, coherent, and humorous. In this example, the young man synthesizes the ego functions of object relations (friendly and open), appropriate affect, thoughtfulness and coherence, and a high-level defense or coping style of humor.

Conscience, Morals, and Ideals

Conscience, morals, and ideals derive from the internalization of aspects of parental figures and social mores. Freud (1926/1959) conceptualized these elements as aspects of the superego. Severe impairments in these functions can interfere with the patient-therapist relationship. For instance, if a patient is not truthful with the therapist, achieving success in psychotherapy may be difficult.

The following case provides the basis for a structural case formulation.

Case Illustration: Structural Case Formulation

Bert, a 24-year-old man with panic disorder, has developed the belief that his coworkers are saying derogatory things about him and want to hurt him physically. His relationships are characterized by an absence of concern for self or others, and this lack of concern often puts him at risk. He uses women to satisfy his sexual needs, abruptly leaving them and giving untruthful excuses. At times he becomes enraged with the women he is seeing and is physically abusive. His aggressive and violent behavior evokes fears of retaliation. He both uses and sells drugs. He has a history of beginning schools and jobs, quitting when he encounters difficulties, and blaming others for his failures.

Bert has impaired reality testing, consisting of ideas about others talking about him and plotting against him. His adaptive skills are poor, as demonstrated by his inability to work or to complete school. Relationships are conducted on a need-satisfying basis, without concern for others. Bert is often sadistic but then becomes self-defeating and self-punishing. He exhibits impaired frustration tolerance and poorly controlled impulses, and his displays of rage may indicate a limited repertoire of affective responses. He uses immature defenses, such as projection, acting out, and denial.

Genetic Approach

The genetic approach to case formulation involves exploration of early development and life events that may help to explain an individual's current situation. The genetic approach follows the development of the child from birth to late adolescence or early adulthood. Life presents many challenges, conflicts, and crises. These events can be traumatic, depending on the severity of the event, the developmental stage of the child experiencing the event, and the quality of the child's support system at the time of the event. Events or conditions important in a child's development include the loss of a significant person, separation, abuse, the birth of a sibling, birth defects and developmental deficits, learning problems, illness, surgery, and substance abuse. Although a single event can have a traumatic effect on an individual, it is often negative experiences in day-to-day life that lead to significant conflict, psychopathology, and characterological problems. Examples of negative day-to-day events include constant criticism, devaluing and abusive behavior of parents, parental conflict, and significant parental psychiatric problems.

An example of a persistent difficulty or traumatic situation is the experience of a young boy growing up with a violent alcoholic father who is demeaning and at times physically abusive. Persistent trauma such as that caused by unresponsiveness of a parent may be more subtle and difficult to evaluate. For instance, a narcissistic mother may use her daughter for her own self-enhancement. She may ignore her child's real qualities, demanding behavior that the child is unable to deliver or can deliver only at considerable cost to herself.

Dynamic Approach

The dynamic approach is useful with mental and/or emotional tensions that may be conscious or unconscious. The therapist using this approach focuses on conflicting wishes, needs, or feelings and their meanings. In a conflict situation, an individual wards off or defends against wishes, needs, or feelings. The dynamic approach highlights the content of an individual's current conflicts and relates them to a primary lifelong or core conflict (Perry et al. 1987).

In contrast to structural case formulation, which is based on an individual's relatively fixed characteristics and functioning, dynamic case formulation is concerned with meaning and content. The dynamic approach focuses on current conflicts, whereas the genetic approach focuses on a person's developmental history, including childhood and adolescent traumas and conflicts and their possible meanings. Childhood conflicts tend to be revived and relived in adult life.

A useful approach to understanding the dynamics of an individual, particularly the core conflict, involves mapping central relationship patterns. Understanding central relationship patterns requires exploration of three aspects of interpersonal interactions: 1) what the person wants from others, 2) how others react to the person, and 3) how the person responds to others' reactions. These categories form the basis of the core conflictual relationship theme (CCRT) method, an approach that relies on "narratives, called relationship episodes, that patients typically tell and sometimes even enact during their psychotherapy session" (Luborsky and Crits-Christoph 1990, p. 15). The CCRT is composed of the patient's wishes or needs from others, how others respond (their actual responses as well as their responses from the patient's perspective), and how the patient responds to others. Understanding and using the CCRT method provides the clinician with a central organizing focus. The CCRT method can be used differentially with patients according to their position on the continuum.

The following case illustrates a dynamic conflict as well as its genetic or historical basis.

Case Illustration: Dynamic Case Formulation

Tim is a passive 48-year-old man whose father has become increasingly debilitated and demanding, a state made worse by early signs of dementia. His father often telephones with complaints and demands, even though Tim has been consistently helpful. After these calls, Tim finds himself wishing that his father appreciated him. He becomes ridden with anxiety and often expresses anger toward his wife and friends, later feeling guilty about this behavior. At work, he has become increasingly anxious and perfectionistic, and he worries that his boss dislikes him and will criticize him.

The dynamic explanation is that Tim has ambivalent feelings toward his father, consisting of anger and possibly a wish for his father to die, combined with positive feelings based on earlier experiences. He becomes anxious and defends against these feelings or wishes by displacing the anger he feels toward his father onto his wife and friends. The anxiety serves as a signal of unacceptable feelings. His boss is viewed as an authority figure and has become linked with his father, who is both loved and hated. In general, Tim is passive and avoids confrontation. He fears making a mistake and being humiliated. Tim's wish to be appreciated by his father can be identified using the CCRT method. The response of the other, his father, is lack of appreciation combined with hostility. The response of the self is displacement of anger onto Tim's wife and friends and a feeling of being unappreciated. The genetic basis of Tim's current conflict is related to his childhood experience of his father being both highly critical and concerned and loving. This early experience has resulted in mixed feelings toward his father, consisting of love and rage with accompanying anxiety, guilt, and lack of assertiveness.

Cognitive-Behavioral Approach

Although case formulation has not been widely used in cognitive-behavioral therapy, models have been developed that are helpful in assessing an individual's problems in cognition (Persons 1989, 1993). Cognitive-behavioral therapy is initially directed at automatic thoughts, which are based on core beliefs or negative schemas. Overt and underlying beliefs are closely linked and are expressed as thoughts, behaviors, and moods. Core beliefs are addressed later in the course of therapy. The cognitive-behavioral case formulation model, as adapted from Tompkins (1996), has the following components:

1. Problem list (including automatic thoughts)
2. Core beliefs
3. Origins
4. Precipitants and activating situations
5. Predicted obstacles to treatment
6. Treatment plan

   The description of Tim (see "Case Illustration: Dynamic Case Formulation" in the previous subsection) will be used to illustrate these six components of cognitive-behavioral case formulations. The *problem list* is a complete list of the patient's difficulties and presenting complaints. It includes the dysfunctional thinking responsible for maladaptive behavior and disturbed mood. Tim's mood problems are anxiety, anger, and feelings of guilt. His problematic behavior is his inappropriate anger toward his wife and friends. His automatic thoughts ("I am flawed" and "I will make mistakes and be humiliated") lead to passivity and lack of assertiveness.
   Core beliefs are hypotheses about the patient's self-schemas and views of others and the world. Tim's core belief is a pervasive sense that he can-

not do anything right. This belief makes him especially vulnerable to the opinions of others. The *origins* of core beliefs are early experiences, generally involving parents or parental figures. Tim's core belief appears to have derived from his relationship with his overly critical father. Core beliefs are generally *activated by situations or events* that are stressful or problematic for the patient. The deteriorating health of his father precipitated Tim's current difficulty and brought him into treatment.

Obstacles to treatment should be anticipated if possible. Obstacles in Tim's case might be reflected in the patient-therapist relationship. Fear of criticism can emerge in relation to the therapist and lead to increased patient passivity in the treatment situation. Tim may be reluctant to complete homework assignments because he may fear that the therapist will be critical. A well-conceived and comprehensive *treatment plan* should emerge from the case formulation. This plan should include goals and the types of interventions to be used. For Tim, the goals should include decreasing his anxiety, reducing or eliminating his anger toward his wife and friends, and decreasing his difficulties at work. The interventions should consist of cognitive restructuring of Tim's thinking about his father and relaxation therapy (including meditation) to reduce anxiety.

The Four Approaches Compared and Applied

A number of similarities exist among the structural, genetic, dynamic, and cognitive-behavioral approaches as used in dynamic (supportive and expressive) and cognitive-behavioral therapies. The concept of core beliefs and their origins is similar to the idea of the genetic case formulation, which provides the origins of structural and dynamic factors. The notion of activating events in cognitive-behavioral therapy is analogous to the precipitation of genetic and dynamic conflicts. Obstacles to treatment often relate to the therapeutic relationship, and thus the concept of obstacles is similar in genetic and dynamic approaches. Cognitive-behavioral therapy adds a different dimension to case formulation and the treatment approach, particularly when thinking problems are present. Dynamic and genetic approaches do not involve a major focus on thinking, but the structural approach does include evaluation of an individual's thought processes.

The following subsections provide case formulations and diagnostic assessments of Mary, the patient evaluated in Video Vignette 1 in the "Assessment" section earlier in this chapter.

Structural Approach

Mary is an intelligent woman with limited insight and judgment. Although her reality testing is intact, her adaptive skills are impaired. She has difficulty functioning, caring for herself, and working. Her object relations are on a dependent need-satisfying level. Mary has low self-esteem, a result of early experiences with her mother and sisters and more recent experiences with her husband. Her depression has intensified her feelings of inadequacy. The defenses Mary uses are at the immature level and consist of avoidance, denial, and projection. Predominant affects are sadness and anger. Mary has many negative thoughts about herself and is somewhat impulsive.

Genetic Approach

Mary is the youngest of three girls born to older parents. Her parents did not expect a third child, and her mother considered aborting the pregnancy. Mary grew up with a sense of not being wanted by her mother. Mary felt she was the least favored child compared with her sisters, who were admired by their mother for their intelligence and beauty. Her mother's attitude toward Mary interfered with her development of a positive self-image, resulting in faltering self-esteem. When Mary was 14 years old, her father—with whom she had a predominantly positive relationship—suddenly died. At that time, her mother became less available and more critical of Mary. The death of her father, who had been a source of comfort during her adolescence, may have added to Mary's impaired self-esteem and neediness.

Dynamic Approach

Mary is a needy, dependent woman who wishes to be cared for. The patient's core conflict revolves around her wish to be wanted and cared for by others (mother and husband). When the response of others is to abandon her (father's death), criticize her, or favor others (mother favors her sisters; husband favors his lover), she becomes depressed and withdrawn, with diminished self-esteem. Her wish to be cared for is an expression of her need to feel she has a right to exist.

Cognitive-Behavioral Approach

Mary's problems include depression, interpersonal difficulties with her husband and coworkers, and an inability to maintain day-to-day functioning. Her automatic thoughts—"I can't do anything right" and "I need someone to care for me"—are based on Mary's core beliefs that she is worthless, a failure, and in need of constant support, without which she cannot function. The origins of her core beliefs are her mother's and sisters' view that she was weak, sickly, and not as capable as her sisters.

Precipitants of and activating situations for Mary's difficulties are her separation from her husband and the discontinuation of her medication for previous depression. The obstacles to treatment are Mary's severe neediness and her fear that the therapist will view her as inadequate.

Goal Setting

For patients requiring supportive psychotherapy, organizing goals should be as follows:

1. Amelioration of symptoms
2. Improvement of adaptation
3. Enhancement of self-esteem
4. Improvement of overall functioning

Setting goals in psychotherapy is important in guiding the treatment. Both therapist and patient must agree on the treatment objectives. The goals set within the first few sessions should be viewed as preliminary and open to change. Both immediate objectives for each session and ultimate goals (Parloff 1967) for treatment should be considered. For example, an immediate in-session objective for Mary might be to develop a mutually agreed-on plan for helping her return to work within a short time period. An ultimate goal for Mary would be to promote job stability and improve relationships with coworkers.

Clearly outlined goals help motivate patients and promote the therapeutic alliance as patient and therapist work toward a common end. The goals of treatment should be derived from the patient's problem areas in order to enhance motivation to change and to promote therapeutic clarity. The goals of supportive psychotherapy are different from the goals of expressive psychotherapy, which are symptom and personality change through analysis of the patient-therapist relationship and through development of insight into previously unrecognized feelings, thoughts, needs, and conflicts.

In the past, it was assumed that long-term changes in conflicts and personality could not occur in supportive psychotherapy. Results of studies by Rosenthal et al. (1999) and Winston et al. (2001) have suggested, however, that supportive psychotherapy can produce personality changes in patients on the healthier side of the impairment-psychotherapy continuum.

The goals of therapy should generally be the patient's. In the event of disagreement regarding goals, the therapist enters into an exploration of the problem. In the case of Mary, one of the mutually agreed-on goals was to resolve her depression and to prevent future episodes of depression. During Mary's previous episodes of depression, she stopped taking her medication when she was no longer depressed. Therefore, an important goal for Mary is to continue taking her medication to help prevent future depressive episodes. After the therapist explored the reasons Mary stopped taking her medication and educated her about the risks of discontinuing, she agreed with this treatment goal.

Setting realistic goals is important, especially with patients who have severe psychopathology. Some patients may have grandiose fantasies or magical wishes that need to be modified. Mary had the unrealistic expectation that her husband would return to her, which she thought would solve her problems. Treatment goals should never be regarded as fixed and unchangeable. For example, once Mary's depression is resolved, she may want help with expanding her social network and improving her interpersonal relationships.

Conclusion

Assessment of the patient's problems, symptoms, and character structure is critical for arriving at a complete diagnosis, case formulation, and treatment plan. Case formulation should be comprehensive—encompassing structural, genetic, dynamic, and cognitive-behavioral approaches. We have illustrated this process by presenting a case example from an initial assessment and case formulation of a patient, as well as describing the setting of treatment goals for this patient.

Techniques

4

In Chapter 2, "Principles and Mode of Action," we described the following principles of supportive psychotherapy: 1) the interaction between patient and therapist is conversational; 2) the transferential aspects of the relationship are subordinate to the reality aspects of the relationship; and 3) the therapist relates to the developmental needs of the patient. Rosenthal (2009) characterized these principles, as well as the need to take direct action to maintain the frame of treatment, as *contextual techniques* because they underlie all supportive psychotherapy and are deemed necessary for its conduct. In this chapter, we describe specific techniques (Table 4–1) that are *interventions* (a term often used to describe the actions of a therapist). These techniques are employed to maintain the therapeutic alliance—without which nothing can be accomplished—and to achieve the objectives of supportive psychotherapy (described in Chapter 1, "Evolution of the Concept of Supportive Psychotherapy"): maintaining or improving self-esteem, ego function, and adaptive skills.

Alliance Building

The term *therapeutic alliance* implies that the work of forming and maintaining bonds is intrinsically therapeutic (Kozart 2002). The therapeutic alliance has been demonstrated to be one of the most critical predictors of the outcome of any form of psychotherapy (Horvath and Symonds 1991;

Table 4–1. Supportive psychotherapy techniques

Alliance building
 Expressions of interest
 Expressions of empathy
 Expressions of understanding
 Sustaining comments
 Self-disclosure
 Repairing a misalliance
Esteem building
 Praise
 Reassurance
 Normalizing
 Universalizing
 Encouragement
 Exhortation
Skills building—adaptive behavior
 Advice
 Teaching
 Modeling adaptive behavior
 Anticipatory guidance
 Promoting autonomy
Enhancing ego functioning
 Reducing and preventing anxiety
  Conversational style
  Sharing the agenda
  Verbal "padding"
  Naming the problem
  Normalizing
  Rationalizing
  Reframing
  Minimization
  Modulating affect
  Supporting defenses
  Limit-setting
 Expanding awareness
  Clarification
  Confrontation
  Interpretation

Source. Adapted from Rosenthal 2009.

Westerman et al. 1995). Thus, the therapist using supportive psychotherapy works purposefully to build and maintain the therapeutic alliance. The therapist sustains the conversation, expressing interest, empathy, and understanding, in order to support the connection between patient and therapist. When the therapist suspects that the patient holds unrealistic positive feelings about him or her, perhaps because of transference, it is typically not discussed. Threats to the alliance are always a concern, whether caused by the patient's life circumstances, the therapist's actual behavior, misinformation, or transference. The therapeutic alliance, misalliance, and the repair of ruptures in the relationship are discussed more fully in Chapter 6, "The Therapeutic Relationship."

The beginning therapist may not know where to start with a new patient. It is a good idea to begin by discussing whatever it is that the patient wants to talk about. The therapist must then decide whether to dwell on that topic or to move on to other topics that are more fruitful or important in the therapist's experience. For example, when the patient has recently been hospitalized, medications are a priority topic. The first questions to ask are 1) whether the patient is taking medications regularly and 2) whether he or she is experiencing any unwanted or uncomfortable effects. When a patient does not take medication as prescribed, the physician often accuses the patient of being noncompliant. Focusing instead on unexpected or unwanted effects of the medication helps to transform the conversation from adversarial to collaborative. Later, the therapist can broach psychological issues that might affect willingness to take medication. Possible issues include not wanting to feel overpowered by medication and not wanting to accept the existence of illness.

The therapist should discuss details of daily life with a nonfunctioning individual and should seek opportunities to discuss the individual's adaptive skills. A person with a chronic disabling condition ought to have the opportunity to talk about it. The therapist should make an effort to know how the patient understands his or her condition and what feelings are related to it. The patient may have fears about the future that are not expressed. Depression accompanies many conditions and may be a patient's response to discovering that he or she faces a life of disability or a response to looking back over lost years and family tension.

The therapist should know about the people in the patient's life. Higher-functioning patients are likely to have important relationships, to think about their interactions with others, and to bring up their relationships for discussion. Lower-functioning patients (and some elderly patients) may lead lives almost devoid of relationships and may talk at length about their symptoms or abstractly about their mental problems. The therapist should make an effort to know about family, friends, ac-

quaintances, and coworkers and, in the case of an isolated patient, persons
with whom the patient has even brief contact, such as caseworkers, pro-
bation officers, receptionists, guards, and meal servers.

> THERAPIST 1: Did you have contact with anyone in the last few days?
> PATIENT 1: My sister-in-law called.
> THERAPIST 1: Tell me about her.
> PATIENT 1: She's gross.
> THERAPIST 1: Can you describe her? *(This is a broader and less demanding
>   question than "Why don't you like her?")*

> THERAPIST 2: Who are the people in your life now?
> PATIENT 2: No one. The only people I know use drugs.
> THERAPIST 2: Is there someone you talk to most days?

> THERAPIST 3: You say your son will come if you call him. Does that mean
>   he doesn't come if you don't call?
> PATIENT 3: He'll drop what he's doing if we need him, but to come on a
>   Sunday afternoon? Forget it.

> THERAPIST 4: Tell me about the people who live in the residence.

> THERAPIST 5: Girlfriend? Is this someone you've known for some time?

Some well-spoken or well-educated patients ruminate endlessly and un-
productively about their introspections and their speculations about the
childhood origins of their trouble, without ever saying a word about their
current activity or the people in their lives.

Esteem Building

The supportive techniques of praise, reassurance, and encouragement are
directed primarily to self-esteem concerns. Through his or her attitude,
the therapist conveys acceptance, respect, and interest in the patient.

Praise

A good supportive technique is to express praise when the patient has accomplished something. Praise can be interspersed throughout a conversation, sprinkled in like salt from a saltshaker. Praise may reinforce the
patient's accomplishments or improvement in adaptive efforts, provided
that the patient is likely to agree that the praise is deserved.

> THERAPIST 1: Telling your mother that you knew you had been rude was
>   a good step. Do you agree?
> THERAPIST 2: You're able to make this very clear.

THERAPIST 3: It's good that you can be so considerate of other people. *(Note, however, that in some contexts, being too considerate may be seen as a symptom, and a statement that the patient is considerate might be presented as a confrontation.)*

False praise or praise that is meaningless to the patient is worse than saying nothing. Falsity and deception are incompatible with any good relationship.

PATIENT: I was always afraid of my mother.
THERAPIST: What were you afraid of?
PATIENT: She came in this morning and said, "Why are you still in bed?" She doesn't respect me. They argue a lot. I was 15 before I realized that she was crazy.
THERAPIST 1: You explained that well. *(This is a supportive comment but, in this instance, false praise. Patient has mixed past and present and his mother's attitude toward him and her relationship with her husband. Thought-disordered responses can be "decoded," but the patient cannot be said to have explained the situation well.)*
THERAPIST 2: It's hard for you to describe these things. You're making a big effort *(accurate and useful)*.

When the therapist expresses praise for something that the patient cannot feel good about, the praise will be ineffective and may even have a negative impact.

PATIENT: I really have been feeling bad. I don't do anything. I manage to eat, but most of the time I'm a blob.
THERAPIST 1: Did you do anything last week besides sit around at home? *(Not content with global self-description, the therapist seeks specifics.)*
PATIENT: Well, I went to a movie....
THERAPIST 1: That's great!
PATIENT: Yeah. *(The therapist does not appreciate that being able to do nothing but go to one movie represents failure to this once high-achieving patient.)*

An important strategy for preventing communication failure is to seek feedback.

PATIENT: Well, I went to a movie....
THERAPIST 2: That was good! Were you pleased with yourself? What do you think?
PATIENT: Not really. It's nothing. I used to be active all day and all night. If the most I can do is go to a stupid movie, I'm in bad shape.
THERAPIST 2: I think it's good that you got out. It's diversion. It's a good step. *(Instead of arguing and making the situation worse, the therapist should have engaged the patient by returning to his bad feelings.)*

THERAPIST 3: So even though you got out and went to a movie, you don't count it as "doing anything?" *(The therapist makes an effort to understand the patient before expressing an opinion. None of the therapists in this illustration were in empathic contact with the patient.)*

Therapists need to find opportunities to respond with honest praise. Too much praise may seem contrived or insincere. The healthier the patient (the closer to the expressive end of the impairment-psychotherapy continuum; see Figure 3–1 in Chapter 3, "Assessment, Case Formulation, and Goal Setting"), the less praise is called for. With patients who are the least impaired, the therapist should express praise only when it is the socially expected response (e.g., congratulations for an accomplishment). Complimenting a patient for persisting with a difficult area in therapy may be useful. Praise coming from the therapist's approval of what the patient is doing is actually opinion or judgment. The best praise reinforces the patient's steps toward achieving previously stated goals.

PATIENT: I took my lithium every day last week.
THERAPIST 1: Good *(judgmental, but appropriately so)*.
THERAPIST 2: Good. That improves your chances for avoiding another episode *(reinforces desirable behavior but is still authoritarian)*.
THERAPIST 3: Good. You said you were going to do this—not skip a single dose—and you did it. What do you think? *(The therapist reinforces self-control and discipline and seeks feedback and further engagement.)*

Reassurance

Reassurance is a familiar tactic in general medicine. Like praise, reassurance must be honest. The patient must believe that the reassurance is based on an understanding of his or her unique situation. Reassurance that is given before the patient has detailed his or her concerns is likely to be doubted. When the topic pertains to the therapist's domain as an expert, the therapist must limit reassurance to areas in which he or she has expert knowledge. Therapists can reassure patients about effects and side effects of certain medications, but they cannot reassure patients about long-term effects of a medication that has just come on the market. Therapists can say, when true, that no side effects have been reported. It is correct to say that most people recover from an acute episode of psychosis within a few weeks or that most people recover from bereavement within a year or so, but it is never correct to say that a treatment is certain to be successful. A therapist can tell a person with schizophrenia that the disease often stops getting worse after some years and that later, the patient may begin to improve. A physician can reassure a chronic patient that he or she will continue to provide care to the patient because this may be more important than a cure. It is never acceptable to offer reassurance that is simply what the patient (or family) wants to hear. If the patient demands reassurance and this reassurance is outside the therapist's expertise, the basis for the reassurance should be made explicit.

PATIENT: All day long when my son is in school, I'm sure something bad is going to happen.

THERAPIST: You see terrible things on the news, but you know the odds are that nothing bad happens to most people most of the time. *(This is not expert knowledge; it is based on knowledge that comes from general education and popular information.)*

PATIENT: I'm having a hard time finding food that isn't genetically modified. It's dangerous. The people in stores don't know, and I get the runaround when I call the 800 numbers.

THERAPIST: I know a lot of people are worried about this, but from what I read in the paper, there have been no reports of anything actually happening to anyone. *(The therapist knows only what he reads in the papers.)* It's important to try to keep up with scientific studies about this and to keep in mind that in your total diet, the quantity of foods that you worry about may be relatively small.

The therapist's role is to teach strategies for dealing with fearfulness about the unknown, not to reassure fearfulness away. Normalizing and universalizing, for most people, are palatable forms of reassurance.

PATIENT 1: When my grandmother died, I didn't really feel bad. My mother was so upset, but I wasn't. It made me feel guilty.

THERAPIST 1: That's not unusual. Unless there's a very close relationship, children often accept the death of a grandparent as a matter of course *(normalizing and possibly absolving)*.

PATIENT 2: When I came out to my parents, my mother wanted to know what she had done wrong, and my father acted like I was a criminal. I still hate them.

THERAPIST 2: We know that this happens a lot of the time. When your parents were young and forming their knowledge of the world, the experts said that homosexuality was caused by the parents doing something wrong. In those days, homosexuality was classified as a subtype of psychopathic personality. Haven't you come across other gay men who have had similar experiences with their parents and who feel the same way about them now? *(The therapist normalizes the patient's feelings and encourages understanding rather than expression of feeling.)*

PATIENT 3: I know I shouldn't be in this program. I'll never understand Lacan.

THERAPIST 3: Neither will I. *(Using oneself as a standard is risky, but here, the therapist assumes she will be seen as a representative educated person and the patient's peer.)*

Adages and maxims are a form of normalizing.

> THERAPIST 1: You can't make your [adult] children like each other *(reassurance given as an authority)*.
> THERAPIST 2: I don't know of studies, but we know from newspapers, literature, and the Bible that siblings often don't get along *(normalizing reassurance given as an educated person)*.
> THERAPIST 3: There's a saying: "You can't make your child eat, sleep, or be happy." I guess we could add "or get along with a sibling" *(normalizing using a maxim)*.
> THERAPIST 4: I have never liked my brother either *(inappropriate self-disclosure that serves no useful purpose and crosses the boundaries of the professional relationship)*.

Reassuring and normalizing must not extend to pathological and non-adaptive behavior or to opportunistic, hostile interactions with others. The objectives of supportive psychotherapy are most effectively advanced when reassurance is coupled with enunciation of a principle or a rule (i.e., teaching).

> PATIENT: Whenever I go anywhere, I have this fear that I'm going to lose control.
> Therapist 1: You won't lose control. *(Reassurance as an authority is useful but not as potent as reassurance that reinforces the patient's strengths or adaptive skills.)*
> THERAPIST 2: I don't think you will lose control because you have had this fear for a long time and you have always been able to maintain good self-control *(reassurance based on patient's history and reinforcement of adaptive behavior)*.
> THERAPIST 3: People with social phobia always fear losing control, but actually losing control is not part of the condition *(reassurance based on a principle)*.

Encouragement

Encouragement also has a major role in general medicine and rehabilitation. Patients with chronic schizophrenia, depression, or a passive-dependent style are often inactive, mentally and physically. The therapist might encourage patients to maintain hygiene, to get exercise, to interact with other people, to be more independent, or to accept the care and concern of others. Rehabilitation requires small steps. Many people discount small steps, seeing each one as being of no great importance. Therapy with patients who have disabilities calls for ingenuity in identifying tasks and activities that can be conceptualized as acceptable small steps.

> PATIENT 1: I don't see why I should waste time in occupational therapy. I'm not going to get a job painting flowerpots.

THERAPIST 1: Occupational therapy isn't intended to be job training for flowerpot painting. The idea is to allow people to have the experience of staying in one place and completing a task; it's about being able to cope with detail, with structure. It's also, for some people, an opportunity to stop thinking about their psyches or their problems. *(Therapist addresses both the "small steps" element and the diversionary element.)*

PATIENT 2: I'm tired of not getting anywhere. My father is willing to pay and I'm going to start college in the fall.

THERAPIST 2: Before you take such a big step, I'd suggest taking an adult education course at the high school or community college. It wouldn't be all that you want, but it's a low-risk way to see if you can handle regular attendance, pay attention, complete assignments, and feel comfortable with other people. *(Enrolling in a degree program and failing is not effective rehabilitation; it is bad for self-esteem. This intervention might also be categorized as advice.)*

Encouragement is powerful because people want to believe that their efforts will lead to something. Encouragement invokes the world of childhood; much like a parent, the therapist can offer specific encouragement that provides the patient with care, compassion, and comfort. *Exhortation* is a more insistent form of encouragement.

PATIENT: I'm eating OK, I sleep well, but I can't get going. My apartment's a mess. And they want me to take one of those "welfare" jobs.

THERAPIST: A demoralized person is convinced his efforts will come to nothing, so he doesn't try. The only way out of it, once you are eating and sleeping normally, is to begin doing things. Any kind of work, even beneath your level, can help you to change your perception and begin to see yourself as a person who can function. Then you can move to something meaningful.

The discussion of encouragement thus far has dealt with only one of the two meanings of the word encourage—that is, "to stimulate, to spur." The other meaning is "to give hope." Therapists also use encouragement to give patients hope.

PATIENT: All I was able to do last week was go to a movie. I must be in bad shape.

THERAPIST: One of the worst things about depression is that it makes you unable to even imagine things being better. If you think of something that was good in the past, it's evidence that supports how bad you are now. That's the illness. It may be hard to believe, but these medications usually make a difference and help the depression to lift. For now, do what you can. Does this make any sense?

Skills Building: Adaptive Behavior

Guiding the patient to better adaptive behavior by employing the techniques of advice, teaching, and anticipatory guidance is a major element of the supportive approach. As stated in Chapter 2, direct measures are used. When the patient is significantly impaired, the therapist addresses evidences of impaired ego function. With most patients, the major focus of skills building is interpersonal transactions. Video Vignettes 2 and 3, featured at the end of this chapter and available at www.appi.org/Winston, illustrate this element of therapy.

Advice and Teaching

Advice and teaching are appropriate in areas where the therapist is professionally expert, such as adjustment, mental illness, normal human behavior, interpersonal transactions, reasonable living in society, and possibly participation in hierarchical organizations. It is important for the therapist to be familiar with the standards and customs of the patient's world. The challenge for the therapist is knowing when to transition from giving advice to helping the patient find his or her own sources of advice and information. Offering advice to a dependent patient can be gratifying but may deprive the patient of the opportunity to grow.

Ideally, giving advice should involve teaching about general principles or methods of problem solving. If the patient senses that the therapist is proposing advice that is clearly not in response to his or her needs and instead reflects the prejudices or convictions of the therapist, the patient-therapist alliance will be damaged.

> THERAPIST: You should do regular exercise.
> PATIENT: What for?
> THERAPIST 1: Everyone should. Obesity is a major problem in this country *(possibly true but presented as a general truth; the patient must infer its relevance)*.
> THERAPIST 2: A number of studies have shown that exercise reduces symptoms of depression. It can reduce the amount of medication needed *(includes advice relevant to the patient's condition)*.

Advice is meaningful to a patient when it is pertinent to his or her needs. Good advice that is not in step with the patient's perceived needs is like a commercial or a sermon: possibly true but not personal, which may damage the patient-therapist bond. In terms of transference, a patient may experience boilerplate advice or false praise as a replaying of a past relationship in which someone on whom the patient was dependent failed to meet the patient's needs. Every therapist should know which of his or her ideas are based on personal convictions or idiosyncrasy.

Advice about activities of daily living is appropriate for the seriously impaired. Advice about daily living should not be given to those who are not impaired, even though it might make their lives better.

THERAPIST 1: When15 you get up in the morning, you should get dressed and make your bed. It's important to have a structure and a routine.

THERAPIST 2: Taking an entry-level job would be a big comedown, but when a person hasn't worked for a long time and doesn't have connections, it's often the only way to get back into the work world. If you later attempt to get back to your old level, it provides evidence to a prospective employer that you are able to do a day's work.

THERAPIST 3: People who are interested in what you do usually don't want all the details. They may be interested to know that you enjoyed a movie, but they may not want to hear the whole story. Try stopping and noticing whether the other person asks a question indicating that he or she wants to know more.

THERAPIST 1: They offer you free credit, but you're better off not getting into debt *(mature wisdom)*.

THERAPIST 2: Let's see if we can work out a strategy about what you should do when you are upset so you don't have to come to the emergency room and say you are suicidal *(adaptive skills)*.

THERAPIST 3: I think you should make a plan to begin cleaning up your apartment because it's bad for your self-esteem to be surrounded by evidence of your inability to function *(rationale explained)*.

THERAPIST 4: If you don't do something about your apartment, it's possible that someone will make a complaint to the health department *(anticipatory guidance that borders on criticism)*.

The therapist should not give advice on issues about which the patient can make his or her own decisions. Abstaining from offering such "advice" is one of the distinctions between psychotherapy and social conversation.

PATIENT: You know I worry about everything. Do you think it's safe to use my credit card on the Internet? I read that they can steal your identity.

THERAPIST: Yes. I've read about that. I think the psychotherapy question is not whether I think it's a good idea but how you come to a decision when there are different opinions or when you have competing pressures.

The therapist can generally provide advice based on what the patient has reported. Providing advice based on surmise, even when the patient seeks the advice, is unprofessional.

PATIENT: My boyfriend humiliated me in public again yesterday. I screamed at him when we got home, and he said I was too sensitive. I can't take it anymore.

THERAPIST 1: Tell him that if he does this again, you're leaving. *(Unless the therapist is totally aware of the unconscious forces that have kept them together, such advice should be left for family or friends to give. If the patient leaves and is then unhappy, she may blame the therapist for giving bad advice.)*

THERAPIST 2: Are you able to talk with him about what bothers you at a time when neither of you is angry? *(implicit advice)*

Teaching is more important than advice. Teaching involves principles, which may be based on technical knowledge or on the therapist's knowledge as a rational, informed person who is familiar with the unwritten rule book of life. The therapist's behavior teaches the patient by example. The term *lending ego* was once used as a metaphorical statement that the therapist's model of reasonableness, self-control, and organization was beneficial to the patient.

THERAPIST 1: You tend to put up with things until you become furious; then, for example, you scream at people. Dealing with a problem before it becomes extreme is usually a better approach.

THERAPIST 2: Even if you are right, people do not like to be told what to do.

Anticipatory Guidance

Anticipatory guidance, or rehearsal, is a technique that is as useful in supportive psychotherapy as it is in cognitive-behavioral therapy. The objective is to anticipate potential obstacles to a proposed course of action and then prepare strategies for dealing with them. For patients who are more impaired, guidance must be more concrete.

THERAPIST: What's your plan?

PATIENT: I'm going to begin reintegrating into society *(nonspecific)*.

THERAPIST: What will be your first step? *(aware that a nonspecific, vague response is not a plan)*

PATIENT: Well, maybe I'll go to the senior center. My son's wife said she'd drive me and bring me home.

THERAPIST: Can you think of any problems that could come up?

PATIENT: She might have to stay late at work.

THERAPIST: What could you do if that happened?

PATIENT: It's near the library. I could wait there, I suppose.

THERAPIST: Good idea. What else? How do you think you will react to being there?

PATIENT: I wouldn't know anyone.

THERAPIST: That's hard for almost anyone. What will you do?

PATIENT: I suppose I could introduce myself to someone who doesn't look too senile.

THERAPIST: Yes. And maybe you could ask the director or someone in charge to introduce you to a few people. People running these pro-

> grams appreciate that it's hard for a newcomer. What if you give it
> a few days and still don't feel good about it?

Anticipatory guidance is especially important with patients who have chronic schizophrenia because they are especially likely to be apprehensive in new situations, unsure of their ability to grasp social cues, unsure of appropriate responses, fearful of rejection, and unable to maintain prolonged effort. This technique is also important for patients with substance abuse, who often fear rejection and may unwittingly invite it.

Anticipatory guidance may be helpful and supportive in contexts other than rehabilitation.

> PATIENT: I'm seeing my internist next week about this indigestion and
> weakness.
> THERAPIST: I hope that you start with the most distressing symptom
> rather than with the first things that you noticed, like feeling tired.
> Are you willing to rehearse what you will say to explain your prob-
> lem to the doctor? And if anyone asks "Do you understand?" and
> you are not completely sure, say, "Would you go over it again?"

Prevention of relapse is an important supportive psychotherapy objective. The substance abuse literature includes practical lists of topics to discuss with patients to prevent relapse (e.g., Marlatt and Gordon 1985, pp. 71–104):

- Identifying high-risk situations and using anticipatory guidance for dealing with them
- Coping with negative emotional states
- Coping with interpersonal conflict
- Coping with social pressure
- Identifying relapse and using anticipatory guidance to deal with it

Little modification is needed to apply these lists to the needs of nonaddicted patients with mental illness.

Reducing and Preventing Anxiety

The supportive psychotherapist intends not only to deal with the patient's overt anxiety (a symptom), but also to prevent the emergence of anxiety, which can exacerbate impairments in ego functioning. The techniques intended to accomplish these objectives include reassurance and encouragement, which were discussed earlier in the section "Esteem Building," because anxiety invariably has an adverse effect on esteem. Supporting or strengthening of defenses has been discussed not as a technique but as a principle or strategy (see Chapter 2). In this section we identify a few of the more common techniques to support defenses. The structured setting of therapy, the *holding environment* (Winnicott 1965), has an anxiety-reducing effect that contributes to the efficacy of all forms of therapy. The therapist models adaptive, reasonable, and organized behavior and thinking in countless ways; this modeling is educational and at the same time reassuring and calming.

The therapist should make every effort to avoid the interrogatory style, which involves asking continuous questions and giving little—the style of medical history taking or the style of a trial attorney cross-examining a witness. To minimize anxiety, the therapist shares his or her agenda with the patient, making clear the reason for questions or topics.

> THERAPIST 1: I want to ask questions that will test your memory and concentration.
> THERAPIST 2: Your relationship with your daughter, you said, was a major worry. Is there anything new there?
> THERAPIST 3: Did you grieve when your father died? Some people have little response and it's all right—but some people who don't have any response have it bottled up inside, and that can be a problem.

Above, therapist 3 gave a longer explanation. The use of extra words, even excessive words, can provide padding that reduces the impact of an intervention that the patient may find difficult or uncomfortable. The supportive psychotherapist avoids forcing the patient out on a limb or requiring the patient to make a stark response. The following two therapists are trying to obtain the same information, but the second uses more words.

> THERAPIST 1: Do you experience sexual stimulation when you see someone being hurt by another person? *(Very blunt)*
> THERAPIST 2: This may seem like an odd question, but it's relevant when someone has a history that involves as much physical conflict as you have had: Do you sometimes experience sexual stimulation in connection with pictures of torture? This could include paintings of martyrs in museums. It's not rare. All those great paintings show that a lot of people have found excuses to portray and look at torture. On the other hand, a person can be involved in a lot of violence and not have this response. *(If the patient says no, he is not in conflict with the therapist because he has been given permission to say no. If he says yes, he is in good company.)*

One of the highly regarded interventions enunciated by Pine (1984) is to tell the patient in advance that something might be anxiety producing. This tactic is effective for minimizing the occurrence of anxiety in treatment.

> THERAPIST: I want to return to a topic that we had to leave once because it upset you. I'd like to know more about what happened when your mother remarried and her husband's children moved in.

The therapist can be even more protective by asking the patient to give permission to go on with an anxiety-provoking topic.

> THERAPIST [*continuing*]: Do you think you can handle talking more about this matter?

Naming the Problem

The patient's sense of control may be enhanced, and thus anxiety minimized, by naming problems. The need for control is one reason why people classify and count things.

> PATIENT: I'm so stupid. I had all those people for dinner, and I didn't allow enough time for the rice to cook, and I thought I was smart to make salad early, but then there wasn't enough room in the refrigerator, and I didn't think to ask everyone if they eat meat. What kind of example am I for my daughter?
>
> THERAPIST: Sounds like this is just evidence of your organization problem. We have talked about it, and you have made progress. Let's talk about some specific things you might have done differently. *(The objective of decatastrophizing is approached by reducing what appears to be a multitude of problems to a single problem with a name.)*

Naming the problem can also be used to meet the familiar medical responsibility of explaining the diagnosis, prognosis, and proposed treatment.

> PATIENT: My mother says I shouldn't lie down so much, but it feels better when I do. I read the ads every week, but the jobs don't pay enough and there's no future. I don't have much money left. It would be great if I won the lottery. There was one job that might have had something, but I would have to commute, and I hate that.
>
> THERAPIST: This has been going on for a long time. You no longer have signs or symptoms of depression, so the current medication seems right. I think your problem is demoralization. That's a condition in which a person is convinced that her efforts will not succeed, so she does nothing. The only way out is to begin doing things, anything. Small steps can lead to small successes. It's a rehabilitation approach. It affects self-esteem and confidence. *(The therapist names, explains, and gives advice—techniques of supportive psychotherapy).*

Rationalizing and Reframing

Reframing or paraphrasing looks at something in a different light or from a different perspective.

> PATIENT: Everything was going well and then I realized I was talking and talking and talking. I've done this so many times. It's as if I have no control.

THERAPIST: But in the past, you didn't know you were doing it and didn't figure out what had gone wrong until some time later. Now you see it when it happens. That's an advance *(reframing—the events are unchanged but given a different emphasis)*.

PATIENT: I was so stupid. I got a parking ticket and I could have been back before the meter ran out. I wasn't paying attention.

THERAPIST: Yeah. That's a tough one. If you figure it's bound to happen occasionally, you can think of a couple of parking tickets a year as a routine cost of having a car *(rationalization—patient benefits from discovering that therapist, who represents the adult world, does not think she is stupid)*.

Rationalization is a powerful tactic for avoiding unpleasant thoughts or feelings.

PATIENT: My son doesn't come very often.

THERAPIST: Yes. A lot of young people are completely caught up in work and home. And you manage to get things done without his help *(rationalization and encouragement)*.

Rationalization is also useful in more expressive psychotherapy.

PATIENT: My son doesn't come very often.

THERAPIST: It sounds like you are disappointed, possibly angry *(hoping to explore feelings of which the patient appears to be unaware)*.

The therapist should challenge a patient's defense of rationalization when it is pathological.

PATIENT: Yes, I bring things home all the time. My husband says it's junk, but I'm saving a lot of money by not buying new things all the time.

THERAPIST: But you told me last time you were here that your husband threatened to leave. Maybe the problem is that you can't control your obsessive-compulsive symptoms *(challenging patient's rationalization that she is saving money)*.

The challenge in use of these techniques is to avoid sounding fatuous and to avoid argument or contradiction.

PATIENT: I feel as bad as ever. I don't think the medication is any good.

THERAPIST 1: You look a lot better to me *(contradiction—not uncommon in physician-patient discourse)*.

THERAPIST 2: People who are recovering from depression usually look better and eat better as the medication begins to work, and this happens before they feel better *(disagreement, but the therapist is conveying expert information that may be useful to the patient)*.

THERAPIST 3: You have to get up and do things. You can't stay in bed all day waiting to feel better *(argumentative and not true in every clinical situation)*.

THERAPIST 4: If you had continued taking the medication as you were supposed to, you wouldn't be in this position *(pedantic)*.

Often, therapists negate what the patient says, thinking that this tactic is useful education. It doesn't help.

PATIENT: I was feeling bad. I was thinking about how I used to get up and go to work every day, and I got good pay. I was a somebody.

THERAPIST: Well, you have social security now *(unempathic reassurance or reframing that misses the point of the patient's situation may have a negative impact on the therapeutic relationship)*.

Expanding Awareness

Clarification, confrontation, and interpretation are useful techniques to make the patient aware of thoughts or feelings of which he or she had not previously been aware.

Clarification

Clarification involves summarizing, paraphrasing, or organizing what the patient has said. Often, clarification simply demonstrates that the therapist is attentive and is processing what he or she hears. Clarification is an awareness-expanding intervention. Both in and outside of psychotherapy, people say things without appreciating the significance of what they have said.

PATIENT: I can't get things done. I have to sell the house, but first I have to get some things fixed, and I don't do them. My ex-wife keeps harassing me with court papers about unpaid child support. I think the medication is working, but it takes the edge off my creativity. She's relentless. I'm bipolar. Don't they have to take that into account? My car broke down again, too.

THERAPIST: It sounds like you're saying that you're overwhelmed.

Confrontation

As a technical term, *confrontation* does not imply hostility or aggression. Instead, it means bringing to the patient's attention ideas, feelings, or a pattern of behavior that he or she has not recognized or has avoided or defended against. In the following dialogue, which is a continuation of the comments presented in the preceding section, "Clarification," the therapist uses confrontation.

PATIENT: I'm living alone in that big house. If I sell it, I can get a smaller place and have money left over, but I just don't do anything. I'm so depressed.

THERAPIST: It sounds like you are avoiding doing the one thing that would provide you enough money to pay your bills and give your ex-wife what she wants. *(The therapist knows that depression is a universally used word and that the patient who says "I'm depressed" does not necessarily meet the criteria for a depressive disorder.)*

Human beings are frequently unaware of significant feelings. For example, in the past, when psychotherapy practice first originated, a patient would often be unaware of what was then perceived as unacceptable sexual feelings. Anger can also be outside of the patient's awareness. Hidden anger may be directed toward authority figures, people who are more successful, those who are manipulative, or those who are dependent and passive. Anger may be the emotional response to paranoid ideation. The discovery of anger does not always lead to reduction of symptoms or impaired function.

Resentment (e.g., of parents, children, partners, coworkers) is related to anger and is often accompanied by guilt or shame. It is often perceived as a negative emotion. For example, being excessively dependent on another person is often associated with resentment. Grief may be a hidden emotion, especially for individuals who do not grieve the death of someone close. Delayed grief may also be present in individuals with schizophrenia whose lives have long been disrupted. After reaching stabilization with antipsychotics, these individuals may finally be able to grieve for the years they have lost or for any suffering they may have caused others. Some individuals are so scared of vulnerability that feelings of intimacy and caring are kept out of awareness. The list of avoided feelings can go on and on.

To simply name the feeling and move on is a supportive technique. When exploring a patient's hitherto unexamined feelings and assumptions, the therapist should seek to learn about other instances of whatever has been discovered. The therapist should talk about the implications of the discovery with the patient, seek to understand the basis for it, and ultimately determine what is to be done about it.

Interpretation

There is no agreed on definition of *interpretation*. Many authors use the term to characterize any proffered explanation of "the meaning of the patient's thoughts or the intent of his behavior" (Othmer and Othmer 1994, p. 87). Others limit the term to a linking of current feelings, thoughts, or behaviors with events of the past or with the relationship with the therapist. Linking these elements is important for achieving the objectives of expressive psychotherapy. In supportive psychotherapy, links between patient and therapist are generally made only when necessary in order to avoid disruption of treatment.

> THERAPIST: You haven't said you disagree with me, but you have found something wrong with every suggestion I have made. From what you have said about your problems at work, it's possible that you do the same thing with other people *(a link between the therapist and current behavior; in supportive therapies, such a link may help with efforts to improve adaptive skills)*.

Insight about historical cause-and-effect relationships is not an objective of the most supportive approaches. Creation of a patient's biography or narrative that makes sense of symptoms and dysfunctions is, however, a useful shared task and often a tactic for reducing anxiety, as stated in Chapter 2.

Conclusion

Supportive techniques can be enumerated and mastered. With practice, the therapist can apply these techniques in many situations. More lengthy elaboration of techniques can be found in a handful of books. Especially useful are works by Novalis et al. (2020), Pinsker (1997), Rockland (1989), Wachtel (1993), and Winston and Winston (2002). Guidance about understanding patients can be found in the thousands of books on psychodynamics and psychotherapy written in the last 80 years and in the literature.

Video Vignettes 2 and 3

Video Vignettes 2 and 3 (available at www.appi.org/Winston) are enactments illustrating the spectrum of psychopathology and the associated spectrum of treatment (see Figure 3–1 in Chapter 3, "Assessment, Case Formulation, and Goal Setting"). Video Vignette 2 illustrates the difficult treatment of an uncooperative patient who has severe, persistent mental illness. Therapy is entirely at the supportive end of the supportive-expressive continuum. Video Vignette 3 illustrates supportive-expressive treatment to right of the midpoint of the continuum.

▶ Video Vignette 2: Severe, Persistent Mental Illness in an Uncooperative Patient

Jerry is a 21-year-old man who was diagnosed with schizoaffective disorder when discharged from the hospital 4 weeks ago. He had been admitted because of self-injury following an argument with his mother. He was referred to the clinic for continuing care. Since completing high school 3 years ago, he has spent most of his time watching TV, playing computer games, or surfing the Internet. He has never had a close relationship.

This is Jerry's third visit to the clinic. The therapist has observed that he is grandiose, that his thought processes are characterized by idiosyncratic connections and assumptions, and that he is negativistic. An important supportive measure is honest praise for the patient's efforts. When Jerry is negativistic and rejecting, he may perceive a therapist who praises him as an ally of hostile forces. The therapist's immediate objective is that Jerry continue in treatment and take the prescribed medication, so her main concern is establishing a therapeutic relationship; she tries to avoid anything that might be taken as criticism and is cautious about praise. She offers advice carefully, with explanations. As often happens in an interview with a new patient who has a significant thought process disorder, the therapist at times does not know what Jerry is talking about. She does not want to agree with anything unrealistic but at the same time does not want to challenge him or ask too many questions.

THERAPIST: So, what's been happening?

JERRY: Not much *(uncommunicative)*. Actually, I just started working. It's a few blocks from where I live.

THERAPIST: Tell me a little about that *(asking for elaboration in general terms; doesn't want to appear demanding)*.

JERRY: It's mostly fixing computers. I started yesterday. It's a friend of my mother's.

THERAPIST: How does it seem after 1 day?

JERRY: It doesn't make any difference *(negativistic and pessimistic)*. It's just like staying at home watching TV. It's really no different.

THERAPIST: What about the fact that you can earn some money? *(trying to identify an asset)*

JERRY: I don't care about making money.

THERAPIST: How many days a week will you work? *(trying to maintain conversation without seeming confrontational)*

JERRY: Well, there's a movie rental business. I'll look after that and fix computers. Maybe 3 days a week?

THERAPIST: OK, so it keeps you busy? *(neutral facilitator)*

JERRY: It's nothing.

THERAPIST: I'd say it's too early to know if it will work out, but it's my impression that you don't want to commit yourself *(clarification without contradicting)*.

JERRY: [*no response*]

THERAPIST: Is there anything about the job that you might find difficult? *(looking for opportunity to attempt anticipatory guidance)*

JERRY: I can fix most any computer. It's usually just that someone's screwed them up *(a positive statement at last)*.

THERAPIST: Right, well I heard that the first thing they told every new computer user was that you can't break a computer *(still trying to establish dialogue)*.

JERRY: They're stupid.

THERAPIST: So you have a job; it seems like you're quite good at this job *(praise)*—but it doesn't give you any pleasure. Do I understand that correctly? *(clarification and asking for feedback)*

JERRY: Yeah. It's just like staying at home, watching TV *(agrees with therapist's perception)*.

THERAPIST: I could go on to another topic, if you'd like. *(The therapist introduces a new topic, "showing the map"—sharing the agenda, asking permission—so that patient will not perceive the questioning to be interrogation.)*

JERRY: [*grunts assent*]

THERAPIST: Let me ask you this: How are things with you and your mother and your brother?

JERRY: My brother is home from school this week, and my mother has been really getting on my nerves. She actually lost her job. It puts a lot of pressure on me.

THERAPIST: What happened? *(conversational response; avoiding narrowing focus)*

JERRY: I don't know. She may have a new job. She might start today or tomorrow. Some guy has to call her. *(The patient talks about his mother, not about his long-standing conflicts with her.)*

THERAPIST: Do you think that she understands how depressed you were when you were in the hospital? *(The therapist tries to maintain focus on the patient's relationship with his mother.)*

JERRY: I don't know. Maybe.

Therapist: Tell me a little bit about the pressure she puts on you *(maintaining focus and seeking specifics)*.

JERRY: Well, I feel like I have to make money.

THERAPIST: So—you kind of think she doesn't get it. Kind of like she really doesn't understand. *(The statement is an implied question—a tactic for avoiding direct questions that might be experienced as interrogation.)* And you know, it's funny—some people, they don't really understand mental illness. They think that you can just sort of snap out of it—like it's in your control how you feel *(an empathic comment and at the same time another implied question)*.

JERRY: I don't try to explain. Some people, when I talk, they listen. Other people, no. I don't bother with them. *(The patient is referring to his self-image as an unappreciated teacher.)*

THERAPIST: Well, you can try again; you never know *(vaguely positive; puzzled about patient's shift of subject from mother to "people")*.

Jerry dismissed the therapist's efforts to reinforce what seemed to be an adaptive step: getting a job. Because the therapist is hopeful that this will help to boost Jerry's self-esteem, she attempts to stay with that topic and refrains from approaching Jerry's conflict with his mother, even though she knows that this is important.

In the next video segment, Jerry makes reference to impairment of sense of self. The therapist deals with this concretely, not naming it as a problem. The therapist's values are in evidence when she suggests that helping people might give Jerry satisfaction at work. She explores the extent of his conviction that making money is wrong—that is, his grandiose rejection of most people's motivation. When Jerry accuses his mother of being "negative," the therapist surmises that this is projection and that he is angry because he wants to maintain his dependent relationship with her.

THERAPIST: What would you say about your mood now? *(**Avoiding confrontation, the therapist elects to start a new line of inquiry—without her usual attention to mutuality.**)*

JERRY: About the same. It's hard to explain. It's sort of like a reflection of where I am. If I'm in a positive place, I can be positive. If I'm in a negative place, I'm negative. *(**The patient's description suggests a defect in his sense of self, an ego-function deficit.**)*

THERAPIST: How's the work environment? Is that a positive place for you? *(**hoping to find a behavior or an attitude that she can reinforce**)*

JERRY: Any place you go where the sole purpose is to make money is negative *(**usual contrary, negative response**)*.

THERAPIST: Even if you're helping people? *(**potentially argumentative—the therapist hopes to find a way to reinforce the idea of work as adaptive behavior**)*

JERRY: I'm not helping anybody.

THERAPIST: What if you worked as a volunteer to help people—you wouldn't be making any money. If it wasn't about money, do you think that would be a negative environment? *(**testing internal consistency of patient's thinking**)*

JERRY: It would be negative at home. My mother would be angry with me because I wasn't making any money. *(**The patient shifts from the therapist's question about work environment and returns to criticism of his mother.**)* When I was teaching English, I didn't charge anybody. But my mother, it would drive her up the wall if she found out that I wasn't charging anybody.

THERAPIST: Well, your mother needs money for rent, food for the two of you and your brother, who's still in school. Don't you think that would be helpful? *(**The therapist's argumentative**)* *question is intended to communicate what she believes are appropriate values.)*

JERRY: It's not that. The only reason she can't get a job is because she's always so negative about everything. Everyone she talks to thinks, "I'm not going to hire this person; this person's going to be a problem."

THERAPIST: How do you know this? *(checking on reality testing)*

JERRY: Her tone, the things she says; it's hard to explain. Just the way she talks to people. It gives the impression that she's a negative person. Everything's going to be a problem. That's why she can't get a job. The guy who said he would call her about the job—she called him, and it sounded like she was the boss. The way she acts, it causes her problems. It's not that I'm not helping. It's hard to help someone who doesn't help herself. *(His helping his mother and her helping herself are not the same, but he uses the words as if they are the same concept; the therapist used "help" to mean "beneficial.")*

THERAPIST: When I suggested that you may be interested in trying to contribute to your family's support, you shifted to talking about what's wrong with your mother *(confrontation, introducing the idea of examining unconscious motivation)*. When you talk about your own motivations, things sort of get fuzzy and inconsistent *(identifying a problem)*.

The therapist wanted to reinforce some aspect of the work situation, but the patient's negative attitude prevailed. He said that his mother was a negative person and because of this had trouble getting a job. Probably, he wants to be supported by her. When the therapist suggested that it would be helpful if he provided money for the family, she used the word help to mean "beneficial"; Jerry construed help to mean improving oneself.

Later, if the therapeutic relationship becomes more solid and Jerry becomes able to look at what he is doing, the therapist can try to show him that mixing different meanings of a word (i.e., a thought process disorder, which is an ego-function problem) interferes with understanding and with communication.

JERRY: What I really like to do is analyze things—analyze my life, the places I go, what I do *(grandiose disdain)*. The result is always negative. I don't see the point of why people do the things they do. I see things in a different way. *I* see things correctly. The way I look at it, nothing I do is really going to change the way things should be. It's like people just decided to live the way they do.

THERAPIST: Tell me, did something happen? *(conversational response to the grandiose statement)*

JERRY: Everywhere I go, everyone's trying to make money. Just look at them. There's no point to what they do. They go to work, they come back from work, they go to sleep; the next day they go back to work *(patient's first elaborated response—about his grandiose disdain for people)*. There's no point. It's not like they're becoming better at anything; it's not like they're evolving.

THERAPIST: I wonder if you feel that you can evolve when you're watching TV *(deliberately argumentative as an attempt to overcome patient's apparent lack of involvement and to encourage further conversation)*.

JERRY [sighs]: I'm one man alone, and I can't change anything just being one person. If I try to do something positive with myself, nothing good is going to come of that because I'm just one person.

THERAPIST: It sounds like you're really discouraged *(empathic clarification)*. If you could do something really positive that you really wanted to do, what do you think that would be? *(hoping to identify an interest with potential for adaptive action)*

JERRY: If I went to college, I would study philosophy—but then where would I be? It's not like I can go to an employer and say, "Hire me; I'm a philosopher." There's no place for people who think about things these days *(therapist missed opportunity to praise his awareness of reality)*. The patients in the hospital—they were more willing to listen to me. They realized that they needed something, and they could get it from me. People on the outside—they don't want to absorb anything. They're not ready to listen to anything. So it was better in the hospital. I could talk to people, and I felt that communication had some purpose.

THERAPIST: It's hard to change people *(tracking, paraphrasing, empathic)*.

JERRY: It doesn't change the fact that people need to change.

THERAPIST: Have you ever thought about the way that you react so perhaps you wouldn't get so upset? *(challenging maladaptive aspect of patient's position)*

JERRY: I think it's appropriate to be upset.

THERAPIST: You've given a lot of thought to your situation—perhaps more than most people—and your conclusion is that maybe you should do nothing because it all seems hopeless *(praise and clarification, tracking)*. It doesn't seem to matter whether your conclusions are correct or not because the isolation you describe usually leads to depression *(avoids abstract argument; gives advice based on professional mental health expertise)*. Everyone needs activities that are good for them—something for their self-esteem—teaching, making money, doing something like that, something that they can feel good about. It doesn't have to be important in and of itself. It could just be something that you like to do. It doesn't have to generate a degree or a career or be the basis of an education *(gives advice and explains the rationale)*. And when I say "something that's good for your self-esteem," I don't just mean feeling superior. I mean something that really makes you feel good. Not feeling superior because you can see the folly in the human condition and feel better than other people *(advice)*. What do you think? *(solicits feedback)*

JERRY: Sounds like a waste of time *(still negativistic)*.

THERAPIST: Well, perhaps you should give it some thought before our next appointment.

The therapist stated her position about self-esteem, making every effort to avoid being critical or argumentative. She did not go into Jerry's portrayal of himself as the teacher whom all the hospital patients wanted to listen to. She explained the rationale behind her advice. Her objective at this point is to establish a relationship based on honesty and openness. In the same visit, she discussed Jerry's use of medications, paying attention to possible uncomfortable effects and to his apparent lack of confidence that anything will help.

Video Vignette 3: Supportive-Expressive Treatment

Ann is a 28-year-old woman whose presenting problem is chronic depression. After high school, Ann worked for several years, saved some money, and is now enrolled at a community college. She has a history of relationships that turned sour. Ann described being sensitive to slights and felt she was often treated unfairly, but she did not seem to have ever been delusional or pathologically suspicious. It was noted at the time of initial assessment that she often jumped from one topic to another, and this was thought to be a manifestation of anxiety, not thought disorder. The diagnosis was personality disorder not otherwise specified and depression.

Ann has been attending the clinic for 4 months. She is reasonably well integrated and has the capacity to think about her mental processes, interpersonal relationships, and the patient-therapist relationship. In this video, the therapist responds empathically, praises Ann's efforts, explains her reasons for questions, involves Ann in setting the agenda, praises her efforts, answers questions directly, maintains focus despite Ann's tendency to jump to other topics, and offers guidance about alternative ways of thinking about what had been perceived as criticism.

THERAPIST: How have things been going since our last meeting? *(the initial question involves reference to therapeutic relationship.)*

ANN: I wasn't so down this week. I got to shop a little bit. But sometimes when I'm there and looking through things, I find it hard to make a decision when there are two or three things I'm looking at *(indecisive)*. And sometimes I realize, "Wow, here I am staring at these things, and people are looking at me and wondering, 'What is she doing?'" *(self-conscious)* But I just kind of push it out of my mind and get over it.

THERAPIST: That's good. I'm glad you were able to get more done this week *(praise, expressed personally)*. Let me ask you—when you had trouble making a decision when you were shopping, did it lead to any problems? *(The therapist elects to focus on adaptive skills.)*

ANN: No. Like I said, I got over it. I was able to sort of move through it. But I guess, since I brought it up, maybe I didn't fully get over it and that's why I'm talking with you about it *(volunteers psychological connection)*.

THERAPIST: What were you buying? I want to understand how this may be interfering with your life. *(Explains reason for question—a demonstration of respect for the patient—which is good for self-esteem)*

ANN: I was buying gloves, and I was just trying them on, seeing how they looked, if they were warm, how they felt. It wasn't anything as ridiculous as trying to pick out the perfect onion to bring home for dinner *(patient is sardonic—evidence of observing ego)*.

THERAPIST: You said you got over it, and then you said you wouldn't have brought it up if it wasn't a big problem, so you seem to be kind of saying that it is a problem and that it isn't a problem. So I'm wondering if you think we should talk about this? *(clarification, then involvement of patient in setting agenda)*

ANN: I think we've talked about it enough. I think we can skip it. I will say that when I got home, I got a call from my mom, and she can really be a pain sometimes. I didn't want to talk to her, but I did for a little bit, and I just told her that I'd been shopping and that I was OK, and I didn't want to give her the full report on my life. I don't know. I don't know if she felt like I was brushing her off. I felt a little bit guilty afterward *(sensitive to potential impact of her behavior)*.

THERAPIST: How did you handle her call? *(Initial focus is on action, not feelings.)*

ANN: I was polite. I told her what I'd been doing, that I was shopping, and that I felt OK. I didn't really spend much time with her. I hope that was OK for her.

THERAPIST: It seems like you felt like you were brushing her off. Were you rude enough to feel guilty? Or did you feel guilty because you didn't do what she wanted you to do? In other words, you didn't want to talk to her **(still focused on action, but adds inquiry about underlying feelings)**.

ANN: I don't think I was rude. Probably it's how I felt. I just didn't do what she wanted. I didn't speak with her longer or spend more time with her.

THERAPIST: It sounds like you were asserting your will **(emphasis on action)**.

ANN: Yeah...yeah, I guess I was.

THERAPIST: That can sometimes be very difficult **(normalizing, empathic)**.

ANN: Yeah. My last therapist used to say that it's all right sometimes to say what we mean, and we can have these ideas that might upset us, but as long as we don't act on them, that it's OK. What do you think?

THERAPIST: I think that's generally true **(direct answer to a question)**.

ANN: Yeah, I guess. I was thinking [when talking to her mother], "I wish you'd just leave me alone. Maybe all this wouldn't have happened—all this trouble that I have in my life—if it wasn't for you." It's *my* life after all. She just really screwed me up when I was a kid.

THERAPIST: You know, you did say that you weren't rude in that situation **(reinforcing acceptable social behavior)**. How do you feel that you handled yourself? **(not revisiting childhood, staying with action and self-perception)**

ANN: I think I was good. I don't think she really had a clue that I didn't want to talk to her.

THERAPIST: It sounds like you were pleased with yourself **(reinforcing good adaptive action)**.

ANN: Yeah, I was. I used to think a lot that things might happen to her, and I'd have these thoughts, and I'd get very, very scared. I would see my mom getting hit by a car, and all these terrible things happening to her, and I would really think, "Oh, these are going to happen." My last therapist told me that it's really OK—these are just thoughts—and that my thoughts aren't going to make things happen, and that I should just relax a little bit about that. And really, my mom wasn't so bad. Maybe I was just too sensitive as a kid. I don't have the same fantasies anymore, but I do get annoyed when she calls. Like I said, I went shopping, and I was looking for gloves, I got some food, and I wasn't really feeling down. That's good. I don't know if it's because of the medication. I don't want to believe it's just all about the medication. I hope it's also something within me and our therapy, but I don't know. I'm trying to get my act together and decide what I want to do in my life.

THERAPIST: OK. You know, you just said a lot of different things. **(The therapist is concerned that patient may have an ego-function problem, i.e., scattered thinking.)** And I think something that's important is to look at one thing at a time. Sometimes when you say a lot of things and you're thinking a lot, it can make you feel more disorganized and more anxious. So I think one thing that's very important is that we kind of take one thing at a time *(explains her concern; gives advice)*. All the things you said could be very important—you talked a little bit about medication, your relationship with your mother, fears when you were a child. There are a lot of different things, and all of them are important, but perhaps we should talk about each one separately, one at a time.

ANN: OK. So, all I know is that when I finish school, I don't want to live around here anymore *(not responding to therapist's teaching)*.

THERAPIST: Do you have any thoughts about what I had said before about your mixing ideas? *(maintaining focus)*

ANN: Oh, about that? Yeah—I mean, you're probably right. Sometimes I know that I'm doing it.

THERAPIST: What about what I said before about jumping around in your thoughts as making you feel more tense? Do you think that's accurate? *(reiterating the point and asking for feedback)*

ANN: Yeah, I think it's possible. And maybe I'll go to Boston. If it's not too big and there's a lot going on, you know, all those schools. Or maybe even to the South.

THERAPIST: How do you think you're going to decide? *(focusing on the process of decision making, not the issues being decided)*

ANN: I don't know. I'll flip a coin. Of course it depends on whether I have a boyfriend at the time, I guess.

THERAPIST: It bothers you that you have trouble with decisions, but from the way you are speaking, it sounds like you are actually able to make decisions just fine. Do you agree? *(Contradicting the patient is generally not supportive, but patient agrees.)*

ANN: Yeah, I guess so. I don't really have to make any decisions now about where I'm going to go after school. I still have time.

THERAPIST: Sometimes when you bring up your uncertainty about the future, it's not really a current problem; it's sort of like you're reciting your flaws. Maybe that's a familiar pattern for you, and you're aware of the fact that you are not called on to make a decision right now *(naming the problem, possibly challenging a defensive pattern)*.

ANN: I don't know. Maybe.

THERAPIST: Sometimes, repeating familiar patterns can be a source of comfort *(education about mental process)*. It's important for you that you don't think you've discovered something new every time you do it *(guidance)*.

ANN: OK.

THERAPIST: Sometimes, when you bring up things that you may feel are problematic right now, they may not really be what your main issues are that brought you into treatment. Sometimes, what the mind does is to focus on these sorts of things, which makes it easier to not talk about some of the more vital issues. I think that it's sometimes easier to think about these more neutral types of things. I'm not saying you do this on purpose, but sometimes the mind has a funny way of doing that. What do you think of that? *(Therapist continues education about defensive styles, being excessively wordy to avoid sounding overbearing; then asks for feedback.)*

ANN: I can understand that. Maybe. I've been described as having a "grasshopper mind." *(Patient agrees.)*

THERAPIST: In some circles, people describe that as charming. And then oftentimes, some people may say that it's a little bit annoying.

The therapist suggested that Ann could alter her tendency toward scattered thinking simply by becoming aware of it, and she provided reasons for being concerned about this behavior. In future sessions, the therapist might, if necessary, look for sources of unconscious anxiety that might play a part in causing this behavior. Whenever the therapist becomes aware of it, she will point it out to Ann and then structure the conversation so that topics are finished before being abandoned. "Say whatever comes to mind" is not the rule for supportive psychotherapy. The therapist praised evidences of adaptive behavior, and she praised Ann's description of her problem, intending to enhance her self-esteem. The therapist did not become involved with the specifics of choices Ann described, choosing instead to discuss the decision-making process.

In the next video segment, the therapist continues with the tentative confrontation that Ann's symptoms served a defensive function. The therapist also tentatively confronts Ann about the possible underlying provocative intent behind what Ann describes as a simple question. In each instance, the therapist is tentative to avoid increasing Ann's anxiety or appearing overbearing because such behavior would be inimical to her self-esteem.

THERAPIST: How are you doing with school? Are you still able to study? *(The therapist returns to current function with a new topic.)*

ANN: Yeah. It's not bad. I get bored sometimes, but it's better than it used to be, definitely. But there is this one instructor in my economics class, and I swear he has it in for me. He asks me questions in class; he's always looking at me. I asked him a question once, and he answered it in a way that showed he thought I was stupid or something. I'm sure it was a put-down.

THERAPIST: That really sounds unpleasant. You thought you were being put down *(empathic)*. And I think this is an important worry—perhaps we can stay with this? *(The therapist wants to maintain focus and also to involve the patient in setting the agenda.)*

ANN: Yeah, OK. Since then, I've just kept my mouth shut, and I'll probably pass the final. But there's something else that's bothering me. I've been wondering whether it's the medication. I wonder if I'm holding back because I am afraid that more is going to be expected of me, and I'll begin to be resentful if I can't meet that expectation. Then I might drag my feet and get depressed again. I just don't want that.

THERAPIST: That's a very complicated idea, and you're quite insightful. You expressed your concerns quite clearly *(praise)*. But something you have to maybe be careful about is almost overintrospecting when you're depressed *(education; tentative, to avoid a challenging approach)*. It's almost like having a pimple that you keep picking at. It can serve to distract you from other issues that are going on and kind of keep you down and keep you feeling quite bad. What are your thoughts about this?

ANN: It sounds like you're saying that I'm being too sensitive, and I should just cheer up and snap out of it. *(The therapist's educational effort was not successful.)*

THERAPIST: No, I don't think it's that way—I think that's superficial. I didn't mean to be sort of superficial like that. *(The therapist attempts to repair the rupture without going into relational aspects of the miscommunication.)*

ANN: OK, so what do you mean? I should just be OK and live in the present? I don't understand. *(Continuation of therapy is not threatened, so transference issues are not discussed.)*

THERAPIST: That to me sounds a little bit like a slogan. I don't mean to be giving you slogans or anything. The point I really want to get across to you is that you feel very depressed, and you are very aware of your thoughts—you're introspective—which can be good, because you have this awareness. But sometimes there's almost too much awareness *(exhortation)*—and there's awareness of negative consequences, and there's kind of a fixation on these negative consequences. There's something called mindfulness *(education)*. And it seems that you are being mindful, in that you are considering your inner world and your thoughts. However, with mindfulness, it's important to kind of leave your thoughts as is—they belong to you—and then sort of let go. And not be too concerned about all the negative consequences and all the what-ifs. Just to sort of step back and be aware of your thoughts without feeling that you have to solve all your problems and act on all your thoughts and worry so much *(expert advice)*.

ANN: Oh, so sort of like, because they're just going to come and go—and I don't need to be so entwined with them? OK, I understand. And thanks for the explanation. I really didn't mean to be disrespectful before.

THERAPIST: That's OK. You know, I didn't really take it as disrespect *(direct response)*. And if it's OK, however, I'd like to sort of switch gears right now and talk a little bit about what happened in your economics class. *(By pointing out that she is "switching gears," the therapist avoids authoritarian style of questioning.)* I know that you had asked a question in class—I was wondering about that *(staying with specifics)*.

ANN: Yeah, so the question I asked was, "Wouldn't it be more sensible to teach economics as a psychology course?" Then I would actually get useful credits for my major. What do you think?

THERAPIST: I read in the newspaper that some important people in economics are emphasizing the social and psychological aspects of it *(indicates source of information that is outside professional knowledge)*. But the question that I think is important for us to address is what your intent was when you asked the question in class. I wonder if on some level you weren't being a little provocative with your question? *(defines the focus of therapy, confrontation)*

ANN: Well, I don't think I was trying to be provocative. I thought it was a good idea. Maybe if economics was in psychology, I wouldn't dislike it so much.

THERAPIST: Sometimes people don't always like to be told that what they're doing is wrong *(education about universals of behavior)*. And even though you did put it as a question, it doesn't mean that you weren't really making a statement *(indirect question about adaptive behavior)*.

ANN: Yeah, but this is college. Aren't you supposed to be able to say anything, to express yourself, to try new ideas in college?

THERAPIST: Yes, you're right—it is college. But also you have to be realistic about this. It's a community college. They're hard-working people who are there just like you, just to learn. They're not training graduate scholars. I'm not so sure it's the best place to bring up a deep debate like the one you had mentioned *(teaches about priorities, reinforces current program)*.

ANN: Yeah. I mean, maybe so. I guess it was just getting off topic, or something.

THERAPIST: Can you buy that? *(requests feedback)*

ANN: Yeah, I do, I understand.

THERAPIST: OK. Well, I do want to stay with this a little longer *(personalizes question)*. What was your professor's response to this, ah, question? *(uses extra words to maintain conversational [not interrogatory] style)*

ANN: He said something like, "That's a novel idea; I don't think they'll do this."

THERAPIST: It seems like you didn't really like that. And I wonder what you didn't like about that answer?

ANN: It was obviously the word *novel*. You know—"novel"—it sounded very sardonic and sarcastic to me. I don't know.

THERAPIST: I understand that, but I think it's also important to be realistic and try to understand where the teacher is coming from,
too. His priority is to get through the class and to make sure
that the material gets taught—not necessarily to engage in a
deeper, more philosophical debate. Does that sound OK? *(education about the rules of life)*
ANN: Yes, it makes sense.

Because Ann's level of integration places her slightly to the right
of center on the psychopathology spectrum, the therapist was able
to employ some interventions that are characteristic of expressive-
supportive treatment, although the therapist's overall stance continued to be supportive. The therapist addressed mental processes
and unconscious motivation, as well as content. The focus was on
Ann's verbal coping or adaptive behavior. At times, the therapist
padded her statements with extra words to avoid sounding abrupt
or challenging.

A few weeks later, the therapist addresses Ann's automatic self-
criticism and raises the possibility that role transition, which is one of
the main foci of interpersonal therapy, is a factor in her discomfort.
The therapist supports adaptive behavior, is empathic and optimistic, and raises the possibility of anticipatory guidance when Ann
speaks of an upcoming date. The therapist supports defensive posi-
tions rather than exploring them.

ANN: Everything is OK, but there is something funny.My English lit
class instructor pulled me aside the other day and said, "You
know, you're better than your grades. You're always making
small mistakes—c'mon, get it together." I understand she was
trying to be helpful, but I went home all sad and down and depressed again, just beating myself up *(automatic thoughts)*
because I know that I screw up all the time *(exaggeration)*.
Everyone has always told me, "Good job; I'm glad that you've
decided to go to college, and you didn't just stay working
some job." But I don't know—I'm thinking I'm in over my head
and that maybe I'm just not going to be able to do it, and I'll
find some way to ruin it again, especially if I slip back into my
depression *(negative thoughts)*. Sometimes I wonder if my
mom hadn't been so critical of me, maybe I wouldn't have all
this insecurity.
THERAPIST: I'm sorry to hear that you had to go through with this, but
perhaps it's not such a catastrophe *(empathic and optimistic
response)*. We did talk a few weeks ago about how quick you
were to see the negative implications of your teacher's remarks and to start feeling very bad about yourself and very
critical of yourself when you looked at his remarks in a certain

light *(follow-up on earlier topic)*. And it also seems like in this situation, perhaps you did something similar. You sort of exaggerated the significance of what she said, and you took it very, very personally—and then you started criticizing yourself. And I'm wondering if you were able to connect the insight about yourself when you began this round of worry? *(establishing that there is one theme and not a multitude of problems)*

ANN: No. I just thought that she was telling me that I make mistakes and that I'm over my head, that it's too much for me.

THERAPIST: *(Because the patient doesn't see the connection, the therapist decides to move on.)* Well, I have a question that may seem a little bit off topic from what we have been discussing. What would you say is the biggest difference between your current life and the way you lived for the past few years? *(gently introduces a new topic—role transition)*

ANN: When I was working, I was always doing things. Whatever I did, I knew immediately what to do—whether it was the right thing or the wrong thing. I got paid, and I knew what I was getting paid for. Now that I'm in school, I have no idea. I take a test, I turn in my exam—I get the grade a week later. Everything is so indefinite. It's not very comfortable. They told me not to overdo it and that I should go along with the plan. And I've been doing that, but if I want something more now, then I feel that I just can't go asking to bring it back. I don't want to look like I'm complaining. I know that school is a good idea. It's been what I've wanted to do all these years when I was unable to do it before, and I had to drop out. It's been my one goal to get back, and now I'm back. But sometimes I just really think that I can't make it. I don't know. I just think, all this time has gone by, and I could have been earning my way since that time that I dropped out.

THERAPIST: I think you put it very well *(praise for being articulate)*. And I think a lot of people would find it very difficult adjusting to a new schedule *(normalizing, education)*. A transition is a hard thing for a lot of people. You were working, and then you go back to school. And that's a big transition *(offering partial explanation for patient's difficulties)*. Now, a lot of change has happened, and you discussed a lot of changes. But it's important to remember that sometimes it can take months to really adjust *(education)*. And just because you're having some difficulties initially with the adjustment doesn't mean it's always going to be that way. It's also to be expected *(reassurance)*.

ANN: OK, so what do I do about it?

THERAPIST: Something you can do is that you can remind yourself when you get discouraged that you're doing something that's very hard for a lot of people to do—you're changing your life *(advice)*. And that doesn't mean that college is too hard for *you* or that you're not up to it—or that perhaps you made the wrong choice. But it's hard and it's normal for it to be hard *(ex-hortation)*. And as far as not making stupid mistakes, do you have any ideas about what you can do—now that you recognize the problem? *(reinforces progress; avoids trap of proposing solution to a competent person)*

ANN: I guess I can just try harder.

THERAPIST: Do you think there is anyone you can turn to for help? *(a question intended as advice to help patient find a solution)*

ANN: I know that in the guidance office, I had seen some material before about how to study more effectively and stuff. It's funny, because when I first saw it, I thought, "How stupid is this?" But maybe I'll just go back and take a look at that again. I think it probably would be helpful.

THERAPIST: So if you look into it, it may be quite useful; it may actually not be a waste of time *(cautiously reinforcing the plan)*.

ANN: Yeah. You know, remember the guy that I told you about before? Well, he called.

THERAPIST: The one who you met at lunch? *(demonstrates that she remembers the story)*

ANN: Yeah, yeah. His name is Michael, and we're actually going to get together this Friday.

THERAPIST: So, what do you think? *(open-ended facilitator)*

ANN: I don't know; I'd like to meet someone nice, and I hope he is. I guess I'll have to tell him that I'm depressed and I take medications. But I probably don't have to tell him that right away. Right?

THERAPIST: That's a good point. Honesty is important; however, the fact that you have been depressed doesn't define you. It's not something you should feel you have to tell him on day one *(specific advice)*.

ANN: Yeah, but if it's going to be something that turns him off and makes him not like me, I'd rather know at the beginning than before I get too involved with him. Then I'll just be more depressed afterward.

THERAPIST: That makes sense. As you said, you don't have to tell him right away *(supports adaptive approach)*. Do you have a plan for this date? *(open-ended question)*

ANN: Do you mean are we going to bed together? I don't know yet.

THERAPIST: Well, I was being more general. I was more referring to any issues you may have about this meeting that you think perhaps we should talk about? *(exploring possibility that anticipatory guidance might be helpful)*

ANN: No.

THERAPIST: Well, during all our meetings, we've talked quite a bit about a lot of things; we've talked about depression, school life, your mother, your past. But there's really been nothing about the men in your life and the past relationships you've had with men. And I know that one of the things you had told me in the be-

ginning is that your depression started at the end of a relationship and that it was quite a nasty breakup *(concerned that
patient's offhand approach might reflect denial).*

ANN: Yeah, it was. No, no—there haven't been any more relationships. Most of the guys in my school are complete idiots. That
being said, I do think I'm ready to move on, and this is only a
date. And I'll see how it goes.

THERAPIST: Well, that seems reasonable. Moving on is a good way to
put it *(responsive praise).*

ANN: I know I haven't spoken about it, but I am worried about my ex.
He has a new girlfriend, and I know that she was in a car accident. And knowing him, he's probably all involved fixing the
car, taking care of her. He doesn't have any money, and I know
he can't afford this. He just gets way too involved all the time.

THERAPIST: Well, help me understand this a little bit. He dumped you,
right—and now you are worrying about *him*. How do you account for that? *(considers exploring what may be the defense of reaction formation)*

ANN: Yeah, that's true. I know it doesn't make sense. I was very upset
at the time obviously, when he dumped me, but I try not to be
mad at people for too long. He hasn't done anything recently to
make me mad. I don't know. I just try not to be mad at people.

THERAPIST: So you're a generous person *(compliment).* Does your
worrying about him affect your ability to do what you want to
do? Most people, when someone dumps them, feel quite angry and quite hurt. They may even take pleasure in that person's misfortunes. Do you think it's possible that your concern
for him is kind of a mask for your continuing anger about the
ending of the relationship? It's funny—that's the way the mind
works sometimes. It doesn't have to be that way, and it may
not be that way, but it is something to think about. *(Use of ex-
cess verbiage is padding to avoid seeming challenging
or causing anxiety.)*

In this video segment, the therapist was able to praise Ann for her
insightful self-descriptions. She instructed Ann about a frequent
source of distress that is an area of major concern in interpersonal
therapy. The therapist did not elaborate but plans to return to the
topic. She did not offer concrete advice about how Ann might try
harder but rather supported the idea that Ann could develop a solution on her own. If Ann had said she wanted to talk about the upcoming date with a new man, the therapist would have attempted
to present several common scenarios to consider how Ann might respond and to explore her fears or likely automatic critical thoughts.
Because Ann did not want to talk about the date, the therapist accepted her choice. The therapist suspected that Ann's concern for
the well-being of her ex-boyfriend might be reaction formation to

mask underlying anger. Had the therapist attempted to go further in this direction, the therapy would be categorized as expressive-supportive; because the therapist did not pursue unconscious feeling, the therapy continued to be supportive-expressive.

General Framework of Supportive Psychotherapy

5

Indications and Contraindications

For years, supportive psychotherapy was described as the treatment for individuals considered unsuitable for expressive therapies—persons who were difficult to treat or for whom expressive techniques were expected to fail (Rosenthal et al. 1999; Winston et al. 1986). From this perspective, supportive psychotherapy was said to be indicated for people with 1) a predominance of primitive defenses (e.g., projection and denial); 2) an absence of capacity for mutuality and reciprocity, exemplifying an impairment in object relations; 3) an inability to introspect; 4) an inability to recognize others as separate from oneself; 5) inadequate affect regulation, especially in the form of aggression; 6) somatoform problems; and 7) overwhelming anxiety related to issues of separation or individuation (Buckley 1986; Werman 1984).

The findings of the Menninger psychotherapy study, however, indicated that patients treated with supportive psychotherapy made greater than expected gains (compared with patients who received psychoanalytic treatments) and may have achieved lasting character change (Wallerstein 1989). In addition, data support the premise that higher-functioning patients for whom expressive treatments have traditionally been indicated respond just as well to supportive treatment. The target complaints and psychiatric symptoms of higher-functioning patients diminish (Hellerstein et al. 1998), and, because of supportive psychotherapy interactions, patients develop a more differentiated and adaptive self. These changes can be measured as lasting reductions in intensity of patient-rated interpersonal problems after termination of treatment (Rosenthal et al.1999).

Studies of individuals with depression suggest that supportive psychotherapy is valuable in the context of moderate depression (Driessen et al. 2016), but studies do not consistently demonstrate superiority of supportive psychotherapy over cognitive-behavioral or psychopharmacological treatment (Arnow et al. 2013). That said, a recent study of individuals with depression revealed a strong preference for supportive psychotherapy over cognitive-behavioral therapy and psychodynamic psychotherapy (Yrondi et al. 2015). Taken together, these studies suggest that supportive psychotherapy may play an important role for some, but not all, individuals with depression. Similarly, studies of individuals with schizophrenia and other psychotic disorders indicate that supportive psychotherapy cannot substitute for traditional psychopharmacological treatment but is a valuable adjuvant treatment strategy for strengthening overall psychosocial functioning (Harder et al. 2014; Lysaker et al. 2015). Studies suggest that supportive psychotherapy can also play a positive role in the treatment of individuals with personality disorders, such as borderline personality disorder (Jørgensen et al. 2013; Vinnars et al. 2005).

Supportive psychotherapy may have an especially important role in the treatment of co-occurring conditions. An interesting study suggested that cognitive-behavioral therapy and supportive therapy had value in the care of individuals with depression following traumatic brain injury (Ashman et al. 2014). A rigorous meta-analysis found that supportive psychotherapy, as with other psychotherapies, reduced symptoms of depression and improved coping in individuals with advanced cancer (Okuyama et al. 2017).

Findings suggest that supportive psychotherapy not only is applicable to patients for whom traditional expressive treatments are not indicated but can also be used successfully with patients with a wide spectrum of problems and with higher-functioning patients. Indeed, the most widely used form of psychotherapy is supportive psychotherapy with some expressive elements. Luborsky (1984) and others have developed various forms of supportive-expressive psychotherapy that have produced positive results in clinical trials. Supportive psychotherapy may be the best initial approach when psychotherapeutic intervention is being considered (Hellerstein et al. 1994). The therapist should move away from supportive psychotherapy only when there is a positive indication for another specific treatment. There are several indications for which supportive psychotherapy has the best contextual fit and specific efficacy (see also Chapter 8, "Applicability to Special Populations").

Indications

Indications for supportive psychotherapy described in the older literature are essentially a statement of contraindications for expressive treatment. These indications for supportive psychotherapy conceptually fall into two groups, which are not really discrete: 1) crisis, which includes acute illnesses that emerge when the patient's defenses are overwhelmed in the context of intense physical or psychological stress, and 2) chronic illness with concomitant impairment of adaptive skills and psychological functions.

Crisis

Crisis is an indication for supportive psychotherapy among relatively well-functioning and well-adapted individuals who have become symptomatic in the context of acute, overwhelming, or unusual stress. Under other circumstances, persons in this group might be referred for expressive treatment because these individuals have good reality testing, a capacity to tolerate and contain affects and impulses, good object relations, an ability to form a working alliance, and some capacity for introspection.

For this group, supportive psychotherapy is usually delivered in an acute-care or episodes-of-care model. For example, a high-functioning patient developed a marked depressive reaction to the change in her body image after a mastectomy. This reaction was accompanied by a loss of self-esteem, a negative attitude toward her work, and problems with social relationships. The patient benefited from an empathic therapist's psychological support, which helped her to begin to grieve the loss of her breast, her feeling of bodily integrity, and her health. As she worked through her loss, she began to revise her expectations and plans and gradually returned to the usual routines of her everyday life.

The following subsections detail some of the diagnostic and situational indications that fall into the category of crisis.

Acute crisis. Acute crisis is not a diagnosis but rather a general description for patients whose customary coping skills and defensive structures have been overwhelmed by an (often unexpected) event, resulting in intense anxiety and other symptoms (Dewald 1994). Crisis is the state that individuals experience when they are faced with actual, impending, or possible loss, such as a life-threatening illness, loss of liberty for a criminal offense, loss of personal or public safety (e.g., after the terrorist attacks of September 11, 2001; after devastating hurricanes and flooding), or loss of a loved one. (For a more complete discussion, see Chapter 7, "Crisis Intervention.") Supportive techniques may even be implemented in the middle of expressive therapies when there is a crisis for which support is clinically indicated.

Adjustment disorders in relatively well-compensated people. People in crisis may meet criteria for an adjustment disorder. Adjustment disorders are time limited, lasting no more than 6 months (American Psychiatric Association 2013a). Supportive psychotherapy can help a patient to manage uncomfortable feeling states and improve or develop coping strategies during the episode. The focus of treatment is 1) to reassure the patient that symptoms are time limited, 2) to reduce stress by clarifying and providing information about what the patient is having difficulty adjusting to, and 3) to support novel coping and problem-solving methods, including environmental change (Misch 2000). At its best, supportive psychotherapy facilitates a more rapid diminution in symptoms and resolution of the episode of illness. In addition, the treatment may help prevent the condition from becoming chronic.

Medical illness. For a large number of medical conditions, supportive psychotherapy is the only treatment recommended. An understanding of the individual's innate defensive, cognitive, and interpersonal styles (i.e., core character and personality) enables the therapist to assist the patient in developing better coping strategies (Bronheim et al. 1998). Supportive or supportive-expressive psychotherapy has been recommended for or has shown utility in the following areas: reducing pain intensity and interference with normal work, sleep, and enjoyment of life in patients with HIV-related neuropathic pain (Evans et al. 2003); reducing the frequency and impact of stressful events in patients with primary (Hunter et al. 1996) or metastatic (Classen et al. 2001) breast cancer; and treating HIV-positive patients with depression (Markowitz et al. 1995), patients with pancreatic cancer (Alter 1996), cancer patients with depression (Massie and Holland 1990; Okuyama et al. 2017) or chronic pain (Thomas and Weiss 2000), and hospitalized patients with somatization disorder (Quality Assurance Project 1985).

Substance use disorders. Early in the treatment of substance dependence, the therapist focuses on development of a therapeutic alliance, both to assist treatment retention and to create a context within which the patient can begin cognitive and motivational work to assist recovery efforts (O'Malley et al. 1992). Kaufman and Reoux (1988) suggested that for patients with substance dependence, expressive therapies (when appropriate) should not commence until the patient has implemented a concrete method of maintaining sobriety because expressive therapies provoke anxiety that may trigger relapse. A broader discussion of substance use disorders is found in Chapter 8.

Acute bereavement. Acute bereavement is profoundly difficult and can overwhelm the coping skills and defensive operations of patients with poor ego strength. These patients generally experience such symptoms as self-reproach, social withdrawal, and an inability to maintain job or interpersonal functioning and anxiety and depressive symptoms such as insomnia and anorexia (Horowitz et al. 1984). Supportive psychotherapy provides the patient with an empathic holding environment in which he or she can talk and vent about pain and hostility, have his or her self-esteem directly supported through reassurance and appropriate praise, gain direction for activities of daily living, and reality-test his or her role in the life and death of the deceased. This process supports the use of healthy defensive operations, concrete assistance for routine activities the patient is not able to perform, and appropriate reaching out as a measure against the tendency to remain socially withdrawn (Novalis et al. 1993).

Alexithymia. Patients who are typically characterized as alexithymic demonstrate characteristics that make expressive therapy difficult, if not impossible. These characteristics include severe restriction of affect, a seeming lack of capacity for introspection, an inability to articulate feeling states, and a diminished or absent fantasy life (Sifneos 1973, 1975). When these patients become symptomatic because of stressors such as acute medical illness, they may become somatically preoccupied and have greater difficulty with coping but remain unable to communicate the effect of the stress on their affective experience. Supportive psychotherapy can specifically address alexithymia by working directly on somatic experiences and personal metaphors and helping the patient to recognize, acknowledge, identify, and label emotions, increasing his or her sense of mastery and self-esteem (Misch 2000).

Chronic Illness

Compared with individuals in crisis, patients with chronic mental illness are traditionally treated with supportive psychotherapy and are more likely to receive longer-term therapy (Drake and Sederer 1986; Kates and Rockland 1994; Werman 1984). Patients with chronic mental illness typically have lower self-esteem related to deficits in adaptive skills and ego functioning. Patients with chronic mental illness include not only those with primary mental disorders with a chronic or intermittent course (formerly Axis I disorders) but also those who have moderate to severe personality disorders and whose idiosyncratic interpersonal styles, adaptive skills, and ego deficits are chronic, pervasive, and maladaptive (Sampson and Weiss 1986). The majority of psychotherapy patients in outpatient psychiatric clinics have probably been treated with dynamically informed supportive psychotherapy.

Some chronic conditions not usually associated with severe mental illness can be damaging to adaptive and psychological functioning and may be helped by supportive psychotherapy. These conditions include later stages of severe medical illness from which the patient is not expected to recover. Supportive psychotherapy has been shown to assist in reducing suffering and in maintaining self-esteem, adaptive skills, and ego functioning for as long as practicable in patients with chronic illness (e.g., cancer; Thomas and Weiss 2000).

Contraindications

Because supportive psychotherapy is based on the factors common to all psychotherapies, it is contraindicated in relatively few circumstances (Frank 1975; Pinsker et al. 1996). Hellerstein et al. (1994) argued that supportive psychotherapy is the appropriate default approach to psychotherapy and that supportive psychotherapy can be applied over a wide range of psychopathology and situations.

Supportive psychotherapy is contraindicated when psychotherapy itself is contraindicated. This list of contraindications is short. Novalis et al. (1993) suggested that supportive psychotherapy is unlikely to be effective in delirium states, other organic mental disorders, drug intoxication, and later stages of dementia; these are conditions in which any psychotherapy would be expected to fail. Individuals who seek help and yet chronically reject all help that is offered (*help-rejecting*) do not make good use of supportive interventions. These individuals may become worse as they repeatedly confirm that the therapist's good will and concrete advice are not useful. Individuals who lie or malinger as a matter of course do as poorly in this treatment as in other treatments. Psychopathic individuals who establish a pattern of pseudomutuality in the therapeutic relationship either quickly understand the lack of opportunity for real gratification and drop out of treatment or become focused on attempting to use the relationship to inappropriately gratify real or imagined needs. In the latter case, in order to elicit the therapist's good will and expected personal gain, the patient may come across as increasingly needy or may become coercive.

There are few contraindications for supportive psychotherapy. A more formal cognitive-behavioral treatment appears to be more effective than supportive psychotherapy for a number of conditions, including Tourette's disorder (Wilhelm et al. 2003); acute adolescent depression (Brent et al. 1997), although cognitive-behavioral therapy does not have a better effect on the long-term outcome of adolescent depression (Birmaher et al. 2000); major depression (Arnow et al. 2013); panic disorder (Beck et al. 1992); obsessive-compulsive disorder (Foa and Franklin 2002); and bulimia nervosa (le Grange et al. 2007; Walsh et al. 1997). The integration of supportive psychotherapy and cognitive-behavioral therapy is discussed at length by Winston and Winston (2002).

Initiation of Treatment

The therapist essentially conducts supportive psychotherapy in the first session with a patient, during which the therapist determines whether or not supportive psychotherapy is the treatment of choice (see Chapter 3, "Assessment, Case Formulation, and Goal Setting"). Supportive psychotherapy is conversational in style and serves as the context for all patient-therapist interactions. History taking, payment negotiations, interchanges on the rules and conduct of therapy, goal setting, and length-of-treatment discussions are conducted within a supportive framework in the first session.

The ground rules of supportive psychotherapy should be made explicit. The therapist should obtain the patient's agreement about the ground rules. The therapist may need to temper the message depending on certain characteristics of the patient, including educational level, ego strength, reality testing, and the context of treatment. The overall idea in creating an unambiguous format for the rules of engagement in supportive psychotherapy is to reduce anxiety by setting clear limits. For example, two clear-cut rules are that 1) no physical aggression and no verbal abuse can be used during sessions and 2) patients should not come for treatment in an intoxicated state.

Office Arrangement

Seating

Seating for supportive psychotherapy is best arranged in a manner that is welcoming, friendly, comfortable, and professional, just like the treatment itself. The therapist should provide adequate lighting that is not harsh and comfortable chairs that are neither too close nor too far apart so that participants can sit upright and see and hear each other easily. Under these arrangements, the therapist can pick up nuances of verbal tone, facial expression, and body language, which are important because supportive psychotherapy relies on a dynamic understanding of the patient. The therapist is sensitive to unconscious communication, even if the therapist does not make that awareness explicit to the patient in the form of confrontation or interpretation.

Physical distance can be varied in response to clinical need. For example, respecting the patient's need for distance, the therapist may sit a little farther away from a patient who expresses paranoid ideation. The therapist should not be too far away or the patient's anxiety may increase because talking face to face with someone for an extended length of time from some distance (e.g., 10 feet) is socially unusual. Sometimes patient and therapist need to be closer than usual, for example, when the therapist is conducting supportive psychotherapy sitting next to a patient who is confined to a hospital bed.

Amenities

In the past, the literature about supportive psychotherapy framed the therapy as a treatment for the most impaired individuals. It was suggested that—in contrast to the abstaining, nongratifying position of the therapist in some expressive treatments—the supportive psychotherapist provide small comforts to the patient in his or her office in the form of a box of tissues on the table or a small plate of cookies or other treats by the door. All psychotherapy should be provided in a humane and respectful fashion in a reasonable setting, and we suggest that this aim can generally be achieved without feeding the patient to enhance his or her positive image of the therapist. Providing food for a patient is concretely accommodating, and although it provides a supportive relationship, it is typically reserved only for the patients with the greatest challenges in functioning. The therapist's provision of practical items (e.g., bus tickets) and snacks for the most impaired patients may help to sustain the therapeutic alliance. Gifts from the therapist to the patient are not expressly prohibited if a gift is related to the therapy, such as an informational manual, or if an institutional practice has been developed to supply items of need to the neediest patients (Novalis et al. 1993; Roberts 2016). In certain cultural contexts, provision of food and gracious acceptance of small gifts are entirely appropriate (Roberts 2016) and always should be acknowledged and explored in therapeutic interactions.

Initiation and Termination of Sessions

The therapist is expected to begin and end sessions on time. This temporal framing is respectful to both the patient and the psychotherapist. In supportive psychotherapy, the therapist does not focus on occasional lateness; however, when a patient demonstrates a pattern of lateness, the pattern can be explored within the supportive framework. In expressive treatment, the therapist labels the pattern of lateness and adheres to the assumption that lateness is due to resistance or other unconscious processes. The therapist encourages the patient's verbalization, with the objective of exploring the resistance and enabling the patient to express his or her wish or feeling, which is generally related to the therapist or therapy. In supportive psychotherapy, the therapist is free to discuss matters of lateness from a practical point of view. Keeping appointments is an adaptive behavior; arriving late to a meeting that is genuinely in the patient's best interests is not. The therapist can attend to such lateness using a collaborative, problem-solving approach. A pattern of missing sessions can be addressed in the same way.

The following dialogue illustrates a supportive psychotherapy approach to lateness.

> PATIENT: Sorry, I'm late again. I just don't know—I was sure I gave myself enough time [*angry*]. No matter how I try, I'm always late to everything! I do everything wrong! I should just go home! *(overinclusive negativism, nihilism, defeatism)*
>
> THERAPIST: I know it can feel that way because it's frustrating to have a habit that gets in the way, but even the hardest habits can be broken [*engaging smile*]. Are you sure you do *everything* wrong? If that were the case, you wouldn't have made it here at all today, and you might have forgotten your socks! *(slogans, humor; challenges the negative self-statements)*
>
> PATIENT: OK, OK, maybe not everything [*begrudging smile*]. I just hate it when I'm late! It feels like someone's got a fix against me, no matter how hard I try *(esteem-lowering experience of powerlessness, projection)*.
>
> THERAPIST: That can't make you feel good about yourself. Perhaps we can look at how you decide what time to leave? Sometimes people leave themselves some extra wiggle room in case of any unforeseen events so that they have enough time to get to an appointment. That would increase your sense of control over things and help you feel better. Want to give it a shot? *(empathy and anticipatory guidance)*
>
> PATIENT: Sure.

Similarly, a patient may establish a pattern of continuing beyond when the session was scheduled to end, which might have different unconscious motivations, all amenable to discussion in the context of supporting ego function and adaptive skills. With some patients and in certain cases, the therapist might determine that extending a session is therapeutically appropriate. For example, when a patient is unavoidably detained by traffic but is in a crisis, the therapist might choose to give the patient extra time if the schedule allows or might briefly connect and reschedule the patient's next appointment if an earlier date is available. Similarly, the therapist is clinically compelled to take a few extra minutes to address "doorknob issues" (Pinsker 1997)—issues brought up as the patient is exiting the session—if they are clinically provocative and raise the therapist's acute concern. Concerns about not gratifying the patient's infantile wishes should be entertained but should take second place to reasonableness, which the therapist should always be modeling.

The therapist might decide not to extend a session because doing so would support maladaptive, regressive behavior without reasonable clinical or environmental justification. Choosing not to extend a session also models behavior for the patient. The therapist must balance limit setting with promotion of autonomy and independence (Misch 2000) (see Chapter 2, "Principles and Mode of Action"). Sometimes, the therapist must get up, open the door, and firmly show the patient out. If the patient continually resists the therapist's efforts to stop on time, the therapist can choose to cue the patient at intervals about how much time is remaining in the session, thus offering anticipatory guidance. The experienced therapist uses these strategies to wind down a session before time is up so that patients are not in the middle of a hot topic at the session's end (Pinsker 1997).

Timing and Intensity of Treatment Sessions

The timing and intensity of treatment sessions should be set through an agreement between patient and therapist, with the proviso that timing and intensity may change on the basis of clinical need, such as when a crisis arises. In expressive treatments, the ideal is to have a constant interval between sessions, which are held at the same time and on the same day of the week, creating a stable frame. Although the frequency of visits is less fixed in supportive psychotherapy, setting a specific, repeated time to meet tends to reduce anxiety. Similarly, the length of a session should generally be fixed but may be subject to variation when clinically appropriate and based on when the therapist can accommodate the patient. Fixed frequency and length bring stability to the framework of the therapeutic interactions.

Phases of Treatment

Beginning

In the beginning of therapy, the therapist pays a great deal of attention to supporting the formation of a therapeutic alliance because the therapeutic alliance increases the likelihood that the patient will remain in treatment and will have a good outcome (Gunderson et al. 1984; Hartley and Strupp 1983). Over the first few sessions, the therapist should attempt to come to a reasonable understanding of the patient's target complaints and presenting symptoms and acquire a working knowledge of the patient's general level of ego function and object relatedness, as well as his or her adaptive strengths and deficits. From these data, the therapist synthesizes a case formulation and hypothesizes areas of acute and chronic deficit in defensive operations, adaptive skills, and ego functioning that should be directly addressed through supportive interventions (see Chapter 3). As the therapist gets to know the patient better, the therapist fine-tunes his or her understanding of the patient's ego functioning and adjusts the intensity of supportive and expressive interventions accordingly. The therapist may require an extended amount of time to develop a clear understanding of the issues of patients who are cognitively impaired because of psychosis, severe obsessive thinking, or mood disorder or of patients who become flooded with anxiety or dysphoria when focusing on certain details during therapy. Once the therapist and patient agree on the goals and objectives of therapy (see Chapter 3), the therapist must consider issues of acuity and timing. For example, after a recent psychiatric hospitalization for psychosis, a patient arrives in therapy wanting to talk about whether he should return to college in the fall. The therapist's clinical understanding is that the patient must secure a stable and structured environment in which to live so that he can plan his near-term future appropriately. Without that stability, the patient runs the risk of increased stress, disorganization, and decompensation. However, the patient has brought up neither the imminent loss of his housing nor his plans to deal with that loss. The therapist understands, before the patient does, the need to address issues in a different order.

Allowing the patient to "see the map" before exploring the territory is an important supportive approach that reduces anxiety and emphasizes that therapy is a rational and collaborative process (Rosenthal 2002). The therapist can explain how the topic about to be discussed is specifically connected to self-esteem, to a specified ego function, or to a specified adaptive skill for dealing with psychiatric symptoms or general social interaction. Such explanation is also consistent with motivational interviewing approaches, in that the therapist asks the patient's permission before giving direct advice or prescribing solutions to problems (Rollnick and Miller 1995). The therapist must accept that at times, however, the patient will reject the proposed agenda.

Middle

The therapeutic alliance usually functions as a foundation for treatment in supportive psychotherapy rather than as the vehicle for change (Hellerstein et al. 1998). The therapist continues to monitor the alliance with the patient during the course of treatment and attempts to optimize the alliance by continuing to use the same attention as in the initial phase of treatment. This therapeutic attunement to the patient contributes to the patient's experience of being understood and supported by the therapist. In the middle phase of therapy, if therapy is proceeding well, the patient begins to accept that the therapist is truly capable of understanding and supporting him or her, and this acceptance can serve as a corrective emotional experience.

Positive transference and regard for the therapist are allowed to accumulate unless they become grossly pathological.

In supportive treatment, the middle stage can and often does go on indefinitely, especially with patients for whom support helps to maintain adaptive skills or ego functions. During the course of treatment, new intermediate goals may arise for the patient in the context of life events or increases in adaptive function. An increase in a patient's adaptive function presents an opportunity for the therapist to review goals and to offer praise for meeting goals, as well as an opportunity to offer the patient reassurance and other support for self-esteem regarding goals that have not been accomplished.

In supportive psychotherapy, the therapist can use well-structured psychoeducational and skills-building interventions and can encourage the patient to pursue his or her interests and initiatives. The therapist can present expert knowledge about the patient's disorder and its effect on functioning in order to increase awareness so that the patient's decisions are better informed. The supportive psychotherapist uses these kinds of educational interventions early and frequently when working with patients living with addiction, which may increase patients' motivation for behavioral change. If the patient arrives with a pressing agenda in relation to an acute interpersonal conflict or an inner need, the supportive therapist can shift the balance from therapist-directed to patient-directed processes, keeping both the patient's goals and the therapist's objectives in mind.

Termination

A formal termination process is not part of supportive psychotherapy. Therapy ends when the goals of treatment have been reached or when the patient elects not to continue. If the therapist believes that the patient's decision to stop is a product of ego-function disturbance (e.g., grandiosity), symptoms (e.g., hopelessness), or faulty adaptive skills (e.g., inability to manage regular visits), the therapist attempts, without arguing, to explore the problem. Even when the therapist has a psychodynamic hypothesis about the patient's motivation, the therapist must balance this hypothesis against the principle that the patient is free to stop when he or she wishes. Therapy may also terminate because of external factors, such as relocation or another life event that forces an end to the current scope of work.

At the end of formal treatment, gains are summarized and an agenda is articulated for the patient's continued work without regular visits to the therapist. An important part of concluding treatment is for the patient to reflect on and celebrate important milestones that he or she has achieved (Rosenthal 2002).

Supportive psychotherapy differs from expressive treatment with regard to termination. In supportive psychotherapy, the patient and therapist do not work through their relationship and the patient is not asked to mourn the loss of an important object or work through ambivalent feelings (Rosenthal 2002). Because constant, positively held objects are frequently too few in the lives of many patients in supportive psychotherapy, the therapist does not encourage the patient to let go of the relationship, which is based on the real relationship and not on transference.

The analogy of school is useful for supportive psychotherapy. The teacher works in the school even when the student is not enrolled in classes; likewise, the therapist continues to work even when a particular patient has moved on from treatment. The patient's treatment can be framed as an organized set of courses, each with a beginning, middle, and end. When the patient's goals are achieved, the course of treatment is concluded. Just as the student who has a worthwhile experience may return for more courses (Pinsker and Rosenthal 1988), the patient is always told that he or she can return if the need arises.

Long-Term Versus Brief Psychotherapy

For patients with chronic mental disorders for whom supportive psychotherapy is primarily aimed at maintaining adaptive and ego functioning toward overall health and well-being, treatment is likely to be framed as an ongoing relationship without a time limit unless constrained by external factors, such as the patient's financial resources, insurance coverage, or continued-stay criteria in a mental health clinic. Treatment does not need to go on interminably if the goals of therapy have been met.

Brief therapy is typically indicated when the psychopathology is expected to be time limited, such as when the patient has an adjustment disorder or a terminal illness, or when an acute loss or crisis overwhelms a patient's defenses and he or she becomes symptomatic. In supportive psychotherapy, the model of treatment does not focus on character change through emotional insight, so treatment is complete not when core conflicts have been resolved but rather when symptoms have been reduced to comfortable levels or when more competent coping strategies have been developed. A patient may return for more treatment when in a crisis or in order to strengthen failing defensive operations or in order to work on something new.

Professional Boundaries

The therapist guides the dialogue with the patient's therapeutic needs in mind. The therapist never takes a turn to discuss his or her own needs. The dialogue is conversational to reduce awkward, anxiety-provoking silences. The therapist's empathic relatedness allows him or her to know when silence will make the patient withdraw and feel overwhelmed and when his or her quietness will allow the patient to manifest an important affective response, as shown in the following examples.

> PATIENT 1 [*after a long pause, a tentative smile*]: Boy, it's been raining non-stop for so long.
> THERAPIST 1: Sure has! Isn't it interesting? Folks often chat about the weather when they're not sure what else they have in common to talk about. It's kind of neat—there's always going to be weather. I wonder if you'd like to talk about how all that rain has affected you, but we can also discuss strategies to talk with people; you told me that's been a problem **(normalizing, generalizing, collaborating, anticipatory guidance)**.

> PATIENT 2 [*after a long pause, tears well up*]: I can't believe she's really gone.
> THERAPIST 2: [*silent*] **(attentive, quiet; empathic concern)**

In expressive treatment, to prevent gratification of the patient's wishes and to promote elaboration of transference material, the therapist typically avoids self-disclosure of any sort. In supportive psychotherapy, the therapist may judiciously disclose personal information to the patient in a purposeful and supportive manner. The paradigmatic model of therapeutic self-disclosure is found in Alcoholics Anonymous and other self-help groups, in which a speaker's lived experience becomes an object lesson for listeners seeking support for their recovery efforts. Many reports on individual behavioral, cognitive, and cognitive-behavioral therapies suggest that deliberate self-disclosure can be clinically useful (Psychopathology Committee of the Group for the Advancement of Psychiatry 2001). Simon (1988) observed that therapists' decisions about deliberate self-disclosure are generally related to several criteria: modeling and educating, promoting the therapeutic alliance, validating reality, and fostering the patient's sense of autonomy. As a rule, self-disclosure by the therapist is appropriate when it is in the interest of the patient's treatment. If self-disclosure is in the therapist's interest (e.g., when it takes the form of venting, bragging, complaining, or seductiveness), it is exploitation. Information that is a matter of public record is typically the easiest to reveal in the context of supportive treatment. More private information or personal experience requires more deliberation (Roberts 2016).

In supportive psychotherapy, the therapist looks for ways to add facilitating comments or interjections that normalize the interaction and to respond to inquiries in a manner that is both appropriate and technically supportive.

> PATIENT [*after a long pause*]: I was thinking, are you married?
> THERAPIST 1 [*if the therapist chooses to answer*]: What are your thoughts about this? **(traditional expressive psychotherapy–style response)**

THERAPIST 2: Yes, I am. I noticed you seemed to think a while before you asked me. Was it a little uncomfortable to think of asking me that? *(empathic concern)*

PATIENT [*short pause, blushing*]: Yes, I thought it might be weird to ask.

THERAPIST 2: One of the rules here is that you get to speak your mind. It's good you were able to ask me, even though it made you uncomfortable. People who are able to master their fears tend to get more accomplished *(praise with modeling of adaptive behavior)*.

At times, a patient will ask a question that is that is obviously inappropriate or extremely personal in nature in order to annoy or provoke anxiety in the therapist.

PATIENT: I know you're married, but do you still masturbate?

THERAPIST: My sexual habits are personal, but we should talk about sexual issues if you are having concerns or problems with sex *(clearly reiterating a boundary rule and then offering the patient a chance to discuss sexual concerns)*.

Patients with more severe disorders may have difficulty at times differentiating the friendly but professional relationship from friendship. The therapist clarifies and reinforces the boundaries in a respectful, nondemeaning way, without being evasive or insincere.

PATIENT: I've got some Aerosmith tickets! So, we could meet at the box office and I could give you one. How about that?

THERAPIST: That's really kind of you. I know that the tickets are special to you, and I want you to understand that I really appreciate that you're thinking of me. It makes me think that our work together is valued by you. But for future reference, I'm not allowed to receive gifts of more than nominal value from my patients. Also, people who have given a lot of thought to these things have decided that it's probably best to keep therapy relationships separate from other kinds of relationships, like friendships, so that nothing interferes.

PATIENT: Ah, c'mon, doc. It's just a concert ticket! It would be fun.

THERAPIST 1: You know, I was never much into heavy metal music. I didn't like it when I was younger, so I really wouldn't want to go now even if we knew each other under different circumstances *(responds truthfully but evasively)*.

THERAPIST 2: I'd prefer to keep our time together focused on our work, which is about getting things done in a very special and professional way, not about friendship. I'm sorry if that's a disappointment. Can we talk about this some more? *(takes responsibility for the therapeutic boundary but is real and empathic in the relationship)*

Because supportive psychotherapy is more verbally interactive than traditional expressive treatment and because the therapist has more opportunity to be a real figure in relating to the patient, greater flexibility is allowed for moving traditional boundaries. For example, to normalize what a patient is struggling with during day-to-day functioning after losing a parent, the therapist may empathically disclose his or her own pain and loss of motivation during a state of grieving. Although the repertoire of therapist behavior and speech is broader in supportive psychotherapy, with a less abstemious relationship, more opportunities arise for the therapist to use the therapy to gratify his or her own needs and violate the patient's boundaries. The therapist must always avoid the narrow but clear domain of unacceptable behaviors that can exploit patients, including sexual contact, borrowing money, or accepting favors or information from the patient that benefit the therapist (e.g., stock tips, chores, or advice based on nonpublic information) (AMA Council on Ethical and Judicial Affairs 2015; American Psychiatric Association 2013b; American Psychological Association 2017).

Conclusion

Supportive psychotherapy is generally indicated as the starting place for a treatment relationship between therapist and patient and thus has few contraindications. Other forms of treatment are undertaken only if specifically indicated and only with the patient's agreement. The length and intensity of supportive treatment vary according to a patient's need and motivation, and termination does not require working through ambivalent feelings about the therapist. Treatment is focused on real relationships, including the patient's relationship with the therapist, but the patient-therapist relationship should be discussed only when it becomes problematic. Compared with expressive treatment, supportive psychotherapy allows a broader range of supportive behaviors by the therapist; however, supportive psychotherapy is still constrained by clear guidelines about permissible patient and therapist behavior in the treatment setting.

The Therapeutic Relationship

6

Pinsker (1997) and others (Misch 2000; Novalis et al. 1993) described general principles of supportive psychotherapy that are related to the patient-therapist relationship. Some of these principles are listed here and are discussed more fully in this chapter.

1. To help sustain the therapeutic alliance, positive feelings toward and positive transferences to the therapist are generally not a focus in supportive psychotherapy.
2. To anticipate and avoid a disruption in treatment, the therapist is alert to negative, distancing patient responses.
3. When a patient-therapist problem is not resolved through practical discussion, the therapist moves to a discussion of the therapeutic relationship.
4. The therapist can modify the patient's distorted perceptions using clarification and confrontation but not interpretation.
5. If indirect means fail to address negative transference or therapeutic impasses, more explicit discussion about the relationship may be warranted.
6. The therapist uses only the amount of expressive technique necessary to address negative transference.

7. The therapeutic alliance may allow the patient to listen to the therapist present material that the patient would not accept from anyone else.

8. When making a statement that the patient will experience as criticism, the therapist at times might have to frame the statement in a palatable or supportive manner or first offer anticipatory guidance.

Transference: Supportive and Expressive Approaches

Transference refers to the feelings, fantasies, beliefs, assumptions, and experiences concerning the therapist that do not originate in the therapist or in the patient's relationship with the therapist but rather are outgrowths from the patient's earlier relationships, unconsciously displaced onto the therapist. Transference phenomena arise in all therapies, but the role assigned to transference in supportive psychotherapy is different from the role assigned to it in expressive psychotherapy.

In the most expressive psychotherapies and psychoanalysis (one end of the expressive-supportive psychotherapy continuum described in Chapter 1, "Evolution of the Concept of Supportive Psychotherapy"), transference phenomena are of pivotal importance for identifying intrapsychic conflicts, and therapeutic gain is ascribed to the emotional working-through of these relationships. The patient-therapist relationship as expressed through transference phenomena is a major area of focus and engagement, whereas the working alliance or real relationship serves as a backdrop from which the patient's observing ego can peer onto the stage (Figure 6–1).

When working at the supportive end of the supportive-expressive psychotherapy continuum, the dynamically aware therapist recognizes transferences and uses them to guide therapeutic interventions. Transferences are not generally discussed, however, unless negative transference threatens to disrupt treatment. The real relationship between the patient and the therapist takes center stage (see the "Supportive" diagram in Figure 6–1).

Between supportive and expressive psychotherapies, where almost all psychotherapy takes place, a mixture of approaches to transference material occurs. Supportive and expressive techniques can emerge at appropriate times in treatment (Gorton 2000), but both the rationale for and content of transference interventions by the therapist are different in supportive and expressive treatments.

Supportive therapists track transference material but address it only when necessary. Focusing on positive transference material in supportive psychotherapy is generally unnecessary.

PATIENT: Doctor, you always give me the right advice, even when I'm not on the ball or I have some wrong idea. How'd you get so smart?

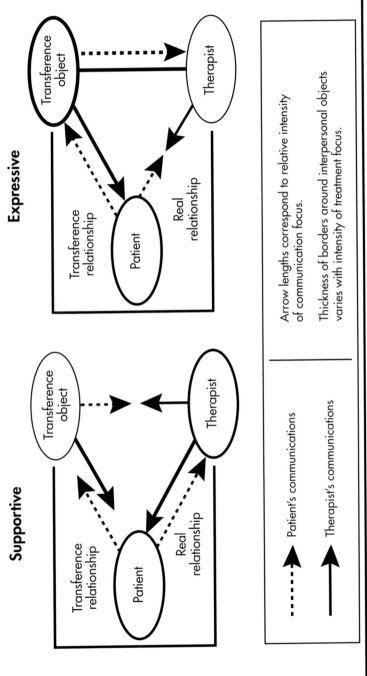

Figure 6–1. Roles of transference and the real relationship in expressive and supportive psychotherapy.

Source. Adapted from Pinsker et al. 1991.

THERAPIST: Thanks, but I can't take all the credit. I had good teachers, and
   I have learned a lot of effective principles from working with patients *(accepts the positive statement but modulates it slightly with
   reality testing)*.

Negative transference is more typically a focus in supportive psychotherapy because such transference can be a threat to the integrity of the
treatment and normally adds to the patient's suffering when acted on outside the treatment setting. In supportive and supportive-expressive psychotherapy, the therapist clarifies often and confronts at intervals but
interprets infrequently, if at all. The therapist's interventions assist the patient in recognizing and addressing maladaptive behavioral or construal
patterns that are reflected in behavior with the therapist; a goal of these
interventions is to increase the patient's self-esteem and adaptive functioning. The patient's behavior with the therapist in supportive treatment
is understood to be illustrative of the patient's behavior with others.

In expressive treatment, transference clarification and interpretation
are important interventions. In this treatment, the patient's characterological and core neurotic defenses are often expressed through positive
and negative transference phenomena. The therapist's transference interpretations and clarifications assist the patient in gaining insight and working through unconscious conflicts; a goal of these interventions is
character change. In expressive therapy, relationships between the patient
and other people are used to illuminate the central patient-therapist relationship.

The content of the therapist's transference interpretations also differs
in expressive versus supportive modes. The precision and comprehen-
siveness of an interpretation may vary depending on the level of the patient's object relations and defensive functioning, the patient's progress in
treatment, and the strength of the therapeutic alliance. Interpretations often resemble clarifications and confrontations rather than interpretations
in the strict sense. Typically, the healthier the patient, the better he or she
will tolerate a precise and comprehensive interpretation without damaging the therapeutic alliance. The therapist can present interpretive ideas
in a supportive manner (Winston et al. 1986). In working with patients
who are more impaired on the continuum, the therapist rarely makes full
interpretations but may make incomplete interpretations (leaving out genetic references and generalizing [Pinsker et al. 1991]) or inexact interpretations (diluting infantile fears with other plausible explanations
[Glover 1931]).

THERAPIST 1: So, keeping your room messy is a way for you to in a sense be
   independent and to do things in your own way in your own space,

as compared with how it is at work, where everything must be annoyingly in its place and on time. Is there a downside? *(supports self-esteem, makes a connection to angry feeling, contrasts patient's style with real-world expectation, opens a dialogue on adaptive skills)*

In the midst of an expressive treatment, the therapist might use interpretation.

> THERAPIST 2: So, keeping your room messy is a way of setting things up, hoping your mother cleans it up. She's supposed to make it OK, and you get anxious about it. Then you become enraged and feel you have little control *(makes a primary connection to a genetic figure and to the role of aggression in staving off anxiety when dependency needs are not met)*.

The Therapeutic Alliance

In supportive and supportive-expressive psychotherapies—for example, brief supportive psychotherapy (Hellerstein et al. 1998), brief adaptive psychotherapy (Pollack et al. 1991), and supportive-expressive psychotherapy (Luborsky 1984)—an early and strong therapeutic alliance (which is reflective of the real relationship) is predictive of positive outcome in treatment and thus is a major focus of treatment (Westerman et al. 1995; Winston and Winston 2002). Because patients with a weaker therapeutic alliance are more likely to drop out of psychotherapy (Sharf et al. 2010), purposely promoting and maintaining a strong alliance has practical utility.

In the early days of psychoanalysis, Freud acknowledged that transference included a personal relationship with the patient, which he called *rapport* or *unobjectionable positive transference*. He considered this relationship necessary to maintain the motivation needed to collaborate effectively and therefore maintained that the relationship was not to be interpreted (Gill and Muslin 1976; Safran and Muran 2000). This view is the earliest evidence of a principle within psychodynamic treatments for managing a strong therapeutic alliance, and Freud's view provides a basis for not interpreting positive transference in supportive psychotherapy. As the concept of the therapeutic alliance began to develop, the focus shifted to the working relationship between the patient and therapist and began to be framed as a *working alliance*, with elements of the real relationship separate from the transference (Greenson 1965, 1967; Zetzel 1956).

Current conceptions of the alliance are broader and include all collaborative elements within the therapeutic relationship. Current conceptions seem a commonsense fit with the construct of supportive psychotherapy (Horvath et al. 2011). The strength of the therapeutic alliance hinges on the extent of patient-therapist agreement on therapeutic tasks and goals, the patient's capacity to perform the therapeutic work, the therapist's empathic relatedness and involvement, and the robustness of the affective bond between patient and therapist (Bordin 1979; Gaston 1990). The patient's perception of collaboration toward a common therapeutic goal may be related to treatment outcome (Cailhol et al. 2009).

The therapeutic alliance is most likely the therapeutic foundation for change rather than the vehicle for change, as hypothesized for more expressive treatments (Gaston 1990; Hellerstein et al. 1998; Horvath and Symonds 1991). The tacit emotional learning that occurs as a result of the interaction with the therapist appears to form the core of the growing therapeutic alliance (Scaturo 2010). Therefore, the therapist fosters the alliance through active measures, acting as a tolerant and nonjudgmental role model (Misch 2000). Direct measures that support the patient's self-esteem further support the therapeutic alliance, which has a basis in the real relationship. The patient may have a fantasy about the therapist's capacities (transference), but the therapist is actively engaged with the patient in a real relationship and is often providing concrete help to the patient.

Misalliance: Recognition and Repair

To promote effective psychotherapy, the therapist must pay attention to rifts in the patient-therapist alliance and make concerted efforts to repair them. In supportive treatment, because the therapist is active, there is greater opportunity to say the wrong thing or to step on the patient's toes. At the same time, to avoid anxiety that might interfere with a positive alliance, supportive psychotherapy does not emphasize exploration of conflict. In the event of a rupture, the supportive psychotherapist has ample opportunity, as well as breadth of strategies, to intervene effectively. Less constraint is placed on the ways in which the therapist might communicate his or her distress at being misunderstood by the patient, as well as his or her sincere regret at having unwittingly impugned or patronized the patient or raised a subject that the patient found intrusive, anxiety provoking, or simply unpalatable. Supportive measures are the first line of repair for ruptures in the alliance (Bond et al. 1998). When the therapist anticipates or notices a misalliance, he or she attempts to address the problem practically, in the context of the current situation, before moving to symbolic or transference issues (Pinsker 1997). The following vignette demonstrates how a therapist addressed a misalliance (see Video Vignette 4, available at www.appi.org/Winston).

▶ Video Vignette 4: Addressing a Misalliance

Rachel is a 35-year-old single woman, a computer engineer, who has been treated successfully with antidepressants for major depression, with resulting increased energy, libido, and concentration. She is typically passive and compliant in her interpersonal dealings and has had difficulty long-term communicating directly what she wants in social and intimate relationships.

Rachel has had several serious long-term relationships with men that demonstrate a pattern of her being too accommodating, with a resultant loss of self-esteem and a buildup of resentment. Because she is passive and dependent, she has often tolerated a significant lack of reciprocity in her relationships, frequently reporting having been "bossed around," yet she stayed in them even when she was no longer happy. Rachel's current boyfriend of 8 months, another computer engineer, is irritable, perfectionistic, and critical, frequently blaming her when things don't go as planned. When her needs and desires are frustrated, she becomes sullen, sarcastic, and full of self-recrimination, which further lowers her self-esteem.

The therapist has been trying over several months to support Rachel in "finding her voice" so that she might be better able to navigate getting her needs served in the current relationship and "make it work." The therapist is using a model of what he deems to be adult behavior in a committed relationship.

RACHEL: I don't know why I'm here [*sullen*].

THERAPIST: Could you clarify what you mean?

RACHEL: All we do is argue, and he never owns up to anything. Just asks me questions, expects me to do whatever he wants, and never tells me what he really thinks. I try to be reasonable, but it's always his way, and it's always my fault. Now it looks like it's over—the relationship's just over.

THERAPIST: I still don't understand. You've described this pattern to me many times before: having a good time, followed by struggling with your boyfriend, and then thinking that it was over.

RACHEL: That's right.

THERAPIST: OK, but I'm unclear as to what you mean by your statement that you don't know why you're here **(attempts, through clarification and confrontation, to get the patient to become more specific)**.

RACHEL: What good is this? I talk and talk here, and now another relationship is blowing up because I can't sustain it. I try to do the right thing, and it doesn't make any difference. I can't do it right enough.

THERAPIST: And?

RACHEL: So, I don't know why I'm here. *(**Again, the patient lodges a complaint about the treatment not giving her what she needs, despite her doing what she believes she is asked.**)*

THERAPIST: We look at these patterns in your relationship so that you can learn ways to change them or learn how to do things differently, which can improve your relationship and your self-esteem *(**indirect attempt to strengthen the therapeutic alliance by reiterating common goals**)*.

RACHEL: Big words.

THERAPIST: I thought I was being clear in talking to you about this, but perhaps I'm missing something.

RACHEL: [*frowns and shrugs her shoulders*]

THERAPIST: You've been working hard the past few months in our work together so that you might be better able to get more of what you want out of this relationship *(**praise for hard work in therapy**)*.

RACHEL: See, you're just like him. I try to do things right, and it still doesn't work out [*looks down, sullen*] *(**states that therapist behaves similarly to boyfriend, with similar impact**)*.

THERAPIST: Are you saying that you see me as having expectations of you here and that when you try to do the right thing, it doesn't seem to work out, and you still feel low and frustrated? *(**clarifies**)*

RACHEL [*nods her head and frowns*]: Yes.

THERAPIST: I see. I've been supporting you in working on this relationship, "doing the right thing," but I think you're stuck in a process that has you feeling down, and not just with him but here, too. And it's not good for you and it's not good for your self-esteem. I can own up to that, and I want to be better able to assist you in our work together. *(**Therapist "owns up" to supporting the patient's staying in the relationship, which the patient feels diminishes her autonomy because the relationship with the boyfriend reduces her self-esteem.**)* If there is a strategy that I'm using that is actually lowering your self-esteem, I'll consider changing it for something that works better for you *(**directly allies with the patient; demonstrates responsive, adult behavior**)*.

RACHEL: You can do that? [*looks up at the therapist, alert*]

THERAPIST: Yes, of course.

RACHEL: That's different from him *(**recognizes a component of the real relationship with the therapist as contrasted with transference or her boyfriend**)*.

THERAPIST: In the past I've supported your attempts on working on this relationship with this man, but you continue to have these powerful disputes where you end up feeling disempowered and blamed. While I can understand your disappointment and sadness in ending it, I do think that you are correct. Staying with this man is damaging to your self-esteem. Here I've been trying to help you to stay and figure out a way to work it out because I thought I had your best interests in mind, but now I think that you know better about your own life. I'm sorry that I didn't catch on to this earlier. Where do we go from here? *(At times, the therapist may have to change his or her position, as people normally do when talking with someone who is becoming angry or distant.)*

Rachel's talk about the relationship blowing up is also a transferential statement about her experience of the therapy and the therapist. Up to this point, she expressed herself as helpless to reveal to him that the strategy was not working and that she was feeling worse. When the therapist discloses to Rachel that he has been using a model that sets up the expectation that she "do the right thing," he sidesteps the transferential bind he may have put himself in with respect to this patient. Rachel begins to experience the therapist differently, such that the alliance is strengthened and she feels that she has been heard.

Resistance

Many therapists might say that the concept of resistance is relevant only to the expressive element of therapy, in which uncovering is essential. However, some of these therapists use the term resistance broadly to signify any patient-produced obstacle to achieving the goals of therapy. In this sense, resistance may be characterized as the nearly universal out-of-awareness fear of new ways and the tendency to cling to familiar patterns even when they are maladaptive. Because supportive treatment aims to support adaptive defenses and build self-esteem, the therapist's strategy in relation to resistance is to increase the patient's motivation for action by encouraging problem solving and new adaptive skills.

Another obstacle to treatment is a traitlike disposition to avoid painful affects, which can interfere with treatment even when the therapist makes every effort to mitigate discomfort or anxiety. In examining the traitlike components of resistance, Beutler et al. (2002b) presented evidence from several studies indicating that measures of patient characteristics typically associated with trait resistance—such as defensiveness, anger, impulsivity, and direct avoidance—are negatively correlated with psychotherapy outcomes. These findings have direct relevance for supportive psychotherapy: patients with high levels of trait resistance tend to have better outcomes with dynamic nondirective, self-directed, or relationship-oriented therapies (e.g., supportive-expressive psychotherapies) than with structured cognitive or behavioral treatments (Beutler et al. 2002b).

"Joining the Resistance"

Supportive treatment aims to support defenses unless they are maladaptive. Again, a primary principle in supportive psychotherapy is to support the therapeutic alliance. When a patient is resistant to looking at dysfunctional patterns, the fact that the therapist reflects the patient's despair and hopelessness or empathizes with his or her tough life or work situation might give the patient a strong sense of being understood and thus increase his or her willingness to work in therapy (Messer 2002). Supportive psychotherapy can provide, without coercion, an active empathic environment and can reinforce the patient's stated goals.

In supportive-expressive treatment, when a patient is struggling to recognize his or her own feelings or impulses, the therapist can follow the patient's lead and make empathic statements about how difficult and anxiety provoking it is to reveal oneself (Messer 2002).

> PATIENT: Mom was usually pretty good about getting to games on time, but Dad used to show up sometimes…usually after the fact. He was always really busy [*looks sad*], and we got along…OK [*pause*]. Hey, you know why I was late today? The cabdriver on the way here—the stupid guy couldn't drive worth a damn! What a joke. How'd he get a license?
>
> THERAPIST: It seems that it's making you anxious to focus on how you really feel toward your father.
>
> PATIENT: This is hard. I don't think I can do this [*tearing up*]. What if I can't do this? **(increased anxiety, self-doubt)**
>
> THERAPIST: Talking about this kind of difficult stuff makes people anxious, but they get through it in psychotherapy. I want you to know that your pursuing it and revealing it here takes courage. I think you're clearly capable of doing it. I wouldn't support your looking at your feelings toward your father if I thought you weren't capable **(empathy, normalization, accurate praise, reassurance)**.

Reducing Anxiety to Facilitate Discussion

Showing the patient a map before exploring the territory reiterates that the engagement is collaborative and centers on agreed-on goals. Anxiety is often diminished when the patient becomes cognitively aware of what is being offered for discussion.

> PATIENT: Sorry I'm late. I started out with plenty of time, but some things came up, and before I knew it, it was 20 after.
>
> THERAPIST: Have you noticed that over the last few weeks, you've come into the session about 20 minutes before our time is up? I feel bad that you may not be getting what you are paying for. Could we talk about it? **(With other patients, the therapist might be uncertain if consistent lateness is related to feelings about the therapy or the**

therapist or if it is due to deficits in ego function or adaptive skills. In this case, the therapist knows from earlier sessions that the patient's lateness is related to the therapist.)

PATIENT: Sure, but I just had stuff to do, and I lost track of the time *(rationalizes, deflects, and plays the lateness off as a result of making more important choices)*.

THERAPIST: In psychotherapy, when someone creates a pattern of somehow getting to the session with only a little time left, it may mean that there is something the person is wrestling with inside that is showing up in this behavior pattern. People do well with looking at what's inside them, exploring it, though sometimes it brings up uncomfortable emotions. I'm happy to explore it with you if you are interested. It might be helpful *(clarifies, confronts, normalizes, offers guidance about the cost of exploring this issue)*.

PATIENT: It's not just here, doc. I'm late for everything [*sheepish grin*] *(generalizes away from the therapy situation but owns the pattern)*.

THERAPIST: So, as a bonus, if we can explore that pattern here, maybe you can learn a skill or a principle that helps you to get along better out there. Is that something you'd be interested in? *(supports motivation, enlists collaboration)*

PATIENT: Sure.

Reframing Resistance as Healthy Self-Assertion

The therapist can address opposition to his or her efforts by framing it as a healthy function of the patient's need for control and self-assertion; the therapist may reduce the resistance by becoming more accepting and authentic (Beutler et al. 2002a).

PATIENT: I didn't ask my mom to enroll me for the spring semester like we talked about last time. I decided to put it off until the fall. I'm just not ready to do that yet. Are you angry?

THERAPIST: It's good that you know your own mind and can make a definitive decision. You must feel some relief about taking a stand. I'm not angry because I don't get to make the decisions about your life, only to look at the decisions together with you and try to help you with how you make them.

Dealing With Distance and Withdrawal

Patients frequently demonstrate resistance in sessions through withdrawal and noninteraction. Because the therapist's verbal responsiveness is a characteristic of supportive psychotherapy, the therapist does not wait for things to unfold if the patient is silent. Silence from the therapist supports resistance and may increase the patient's anxiety. In supportive psychotherapy, when the patient is silent or unresponsive, the therapist selects an issue for attention. The issue may be directly related to the patient's lack of verbal engagement, which the therapist might choose to address indirectly. Alternatively, the therapist might switch to another topic entirely.

> PATIENT: Hello again [*sits down*]. I don't really have much to talk about today [*sits quietly, looking at the therapist blankly*].
>
> THERAPIST 1 [*warmly*]: It's good to see you again. So, can we get back to the topic you were discussing with me before I left on vacation? You were describing how hard it was to follow through on asking for a transfer at work and how those "Why bother?" thoughts were getting in your way. *(The therapist picks up the patient's topic from before the therapist's absence, reconnecting with the patient and supporting the patient's self-esteem by showing that the patient was important enough for the therapist to remember the issue. This approach focuses indirectly on the patient's distancing maneuvers and sidesteps what the therapist assumes are the patient's negative emotions about the therapist's absence and increased anxiety about revealing them.)*
>
> THERAPIST 2: Hello. It's good to see you again. Well, it's been 3 weeks since our last session. Although I had someone covering for emergencies, it's not the same as coming for therapy.
>
> PATIENT: That's right [*looks at the therapist less blankly*] *(engages a bit, reinforces the therapist's coming in closer)*.
>
> THERAPIST 2: Sometimes, when people say they don't have anything on their mind or much to talk about, they actually do but aren't quite sure whether to or how to say something. Patients often find themselves in that situation when their therapists come back after a vacation *(clarifies the situation but generalizes away from the specifics of the patient and the therapist before confronting the patient's denial and withdrawal)*.

The therapist must be alert to distancing negative responses and must be able to anticipate and avoid a disruption in treatment. Not addressing misalliance may lead to a treatment disruption. The therapist must decide whether the situation requires intervention through confrontation or whether indirect means will suffice. The therapist must always evaluate the situation, through introspection, to ensure he or she is not becoming involved in a countertransference enactment (Robbins 2000).

Countertransference

As aptly stated by Clever and Tulsky (2002), "Asking patients to tell us what they want potentially opens an imagined Pandora's box of outrageous requests, and it requires energy both to negotiate this tactfully and to manage the countertransference such negotiation produces in ourselves" (p. 893).

Defining Countertransference

In considering countertransference, the therapist must make a distinction between 1) emotional reactions to a patient's behavior that are due to the therapist's issues and 2) emotional reactions that are the therapist's response to the patient's unconscious attempt to provoke a reaction, which might be a manifestation of transference, coming from the patient's internal world (Messer 2002). The first type of countertransference is what has been described as the narrow or classical view of countertransference—essentially, the therapist's transference to the patient (Gabbard 2001). A broader definition of countertransference includes the real relationship, consisting of reactions most people would have to the patient, as determined by moment-to-moment patient behavior in the therapeutic relationship. On a related note, when the therapist is lacking in expertise or when the type of therapy is not helpful for the patient or problem, the therapist might mistakenly identify his or her bad feelings about the patient and treatment as countertransference, or the therapist might misperceive the problem as the patient's resistance. The therapist makes an attribution that the patient is being resistant, but actually, the therapist or treatment is not effective.

Because we describe supportive psychotherapy as a dynamically informed treatment, the second or broader view of countertransference has a place in our discussion of technical work with patients. This view is that emotional reactions of the therapist to the patient represent useful information related to the patient's inner world and unconscious processes (Gabbard 2001). Currently, many psychoanalytic theorists from varying perspectives hold a consensus view that countertransference is a transactional construct, affected by what the therapist brings to the situation as well as by what the patient projects (Gabbard 2001; Kiesler 2001). A discussion of therapist transference is beyond the scope of this chapter, but it is incumbent on the therapist to attempt to distinguish his or her own feelings from those provoked by the patient or, in the case of projective identification, those that arise in the patient.

Supportive psychotherapy aims to improve adaptive skills. Maladaptive behavior patterns in the patient's real life frequently manifest as countertransference elicitations in the therapy session. When the therapist recognizes that his or her reactions to the patient are the same as others' reactions, sharing this awareness with the patient may be useful in framing practical interventions to assist the patient with better interpersonal adaptation. The therapist must be aware, however, that his or her intent to self-disclose feelings toward the patient could represent the therapist's own needs, not the requirements of the therapeutic situation. Such an awareness is more important in supportive psychotherapy, in which the flow of dialogue is conversational, than in expressive treatment, in which the therapist may at times abstain from responding. Gelso et al. (1995, 2002) demonstrated that better countertransference management correlated positively with better outcome in brief therapy (consisting of 12 sessions).

The therapist in the following dialogue recognizes the patient's maladaptive behavior pattern.

> PATIENT: Everyone always blows me off. I try to be nice—you know, join in, tell stories and stuff—then I see them look at each other, and they throw it in my face, and they make excuses and leave. Like they're so cool. That Andy—he's a piece of work, and I told him so.
>
> THERAPIST: It must be hard to try joining in and be rejected like that *(empathic)*.
>
> PATIENT: Stop talking down to me. Jeez, you shrinks always act like you're Mother Teresa, but she didn't take the money for herself, did she? *(feels impugned, attacks by questioning the therapist's motives)*
>
> THERAPIST: Hmm. It sounds like how you are being here with me is how you've described interacting with Andy and Fred at work. I'm finding my temperature rising with your criticisms of me, and I can't help but wonder if you get the guys at work to feel the same way—except I won't act on my feelings the way that they do. I'll continue to sit and talk with you; I won't make excuses and leave. *(Modulated confrontation and drawing of parallels. The therapist restates her commitment to the process and offers disconfirmation of the patient's expected rejection in spite of the pressure to reject the patient.)*
>
> PATIENT: Oh, sure! Now you're saying it's my fault you're angry? *(continues the verbal assault, feels criticized anyway)*
>
> THERAPIST: I think if we get into an argument, I won't be doing my job of being helpful to you, and you'll keep feeling put down. No, what I'm asking you to do is to see if there's a pattern here that we can work on to help you to get along better with people, because you've told me you would like that *(clarifies; does not get pulled into acting out of countertransference feeling but uses the countertransference knowledge productively by recommitting to the work, focusing on the alliance in spite of heightened feelings, and reinforcing the patient's treatment goal)*.

From the vantage point of interpersonal communication theory, Kiesler (2001) described effective feedback of countertransference feelings as applying the principle that disclosing metaphors or fantasies has the least threatening effect, compared with sharing direct feelings or tending toward action. This principle is highly consistent with supportive psychotherapy approaches, in which it is safer, more respectful, and more protective of the therapeutic alliance to say, "I'm finding my temperature rising" than to say, "I'm so angry, I feel like punching you out." The therapist's modulated expression of countertransference feeling not only offers disconfirmation of the patient's maladaptive construal style but also models adult restraint and containment (but not denial) of affect. The therapist who responds to the patient's hostility in a complementarily hostile way is arguing. Besides being bad supportive technique, a therapist's hostile response is predictive of poor outcome (Henry et al. 1986, 1990).

Handling Devaluation

Being devalued by a patient can be painful and is sometimes a frequent experience for therapists working with patients diagnosed with borderline or narcissistic psychopathology. The therapist adaptively responds and encourages the patient to understand the response as helpful and consistent with the goals of treatment rather than as retaliatory or as a way for the therapist to remove himself or herself as the object of the patient's aggression (Robbins 2000). The therapist must bind the affects and be aware of countertransference responses elicited by the attack, which may include anger over the patient's display of narcissism.

> PATIENT: I needed that note from you, and you screwed up! I left word on your voice mail that I needed it by Monday [*vindictive tone*]. Figures. You could only get into medical school at a state school.
>
> THERAPIST 1 [*feels guilty*]: I'm really sorry. Next time I'll try to be more sensitive to your needs, but I was out on Monday *(masochistic countertransference response to what was actually an unreasonable demand, a mea culpa gratifying the patient's grandiose self)*.
>
> THERAPIST 2 [*feels irritated*]: You're pretty quick to blame me and make critical comments, but you take no responsibility at all for what happened. You left the request over the weekend, and I was out on Monday *(accurate but critical rebuttal, which may leave the patient feeling demeaned and angry)*.
>
> PATIENT: I've heard those excuses before! I needed you. Now, how can I trust you? I knew I should have gone to that Park Avenue shrink my mother told me about! He went to Harvard. He's quoted in the newspaper all the time.
>
> THERAPIST 3: Sometimes I'm going to disappoint you. It happens, even in the best relationships. It might scare you or make you angry that I'm not perfectly attuned to your needs, but fortunately, I don't need to be perfect to be helpful to you. I'll bet that other psychiatrist doesn't need to be perfect either to be effective *(authentic but measured response; models healthy, adult behavior that is neither retaliating nor capitulating; clarifies the role of a "good-enough" therapist)*.

The therapist must have appropriate training and the ability to understand feelings of irritation, frustration, and helplessness generated in response to a patient's chronic criticism and devaluation. Without adequate peer support or professional supervision, the therapist may become clinically disenchanted or disempowered and become either bored or overly confrontational (Rosenthal 2002).

Distancing from empathic connection is a common response by the therapist to a patient's projective identifications (Kaufman 1992). Rather than identifying with the patient's projections and either capitulating or counterattacking, the therapist manages vulnerability and aggression in the context of being devalued. Such management is in concordance with supportive principles (Robbins 2000) and can allow the patient to establish an idealizing transference. The idealizing transference can enable the patient to experience safety in the relationship with the idealized therapist, which can serve as a corrective emotional experience (Alexander and French 1946). Certain patients, such as individuals who seek help but chronically reject all help that is offered (see Chapter 5, "General Framework of Supportive Psychotherapy"), will maintain a transference position that is impermeable to therapist intervention and disclosure. These patients' pathogenic beliefs regarding self and others are confirmed by the therapist's repeated attempts to engage and problem solve (Sampson and Weiss 1986).

Conclusion

A robust therapeutic alliance is a strong predicator of positive outcome in psychotherapy. In supportive psychotherapy, the alliance is posited as the foundation for therapeutic change; therefore, the clinician actively promotes and maintains the therapeutic alliance. In supportive psychotherapy, as in expressive psychotherapy, the clinician observes and tracks transference phenomena, but these phenomena are generally not a topic of discussion or interpretation in supportive psychotherapy unless the impact of negative transference is likely to interrupt treatment. The therapist typically uses clarification and confrontation in supportive treatment, but when interpretations are made, they tend to be incomplete or inexact. Because defenses are not confronted in supportive psychotherapy unless they are maladaptive, the clinician can learn to manage resistance with supportive techniques. The clinician must always be alert to the potential role of countertransference so that it can be properly managed.

Crisis Intervention 7

History and Theory

Crisis intervention began during World War II out of the necessity of treating soldiers exposed to battlefield conditions. In World War I, soldiers with combat fatigue or "shell shock" were quickly evacuated from the front lines, without treatment, despite observations that early intervention might reduce psychiatric morbidity (Salmon 1919). These soldiers often regressed or even became chronically impaired. In World War II, soldiers were treated at or near the front lines with crisis intervention techniques and were quickly returned to their combat units (Glass 1954).

During the time of World War II, Lindemann began working with survivors of the Cocoanut Grove nightclub fire in Boston and their relatives. These individuals were experiencing acute grief and were unable to cope with their bereavement. In his pioneering article, Lindemann (1994) described and contrasted normal and morbid grief. Survivors and their families were helped to do the necessary *grief work*, which involved going through the mourning process and experiencing the loss. One of Lindemann's colleagues, Gerald Caplan (1961), began to work in the field of preventive psychiatry and helped develop the theoretical basis for the community mental health movement. Lindemann and Caplan were among the most important early theoreticians of the crisis intervention approach.

Parad and Parad (1990) define *crisis* as an "upset in a steady state, a turning point leading to better or worse, a disruption or breakdown in a person's or family's normal or usual pattern of functioning" (pp. 3–4). A crisis occurs when an individual encounters a situation that leads to a collapse in his or her usual pattern of functioning, entering a state of psychological disequilibrium. Generally, a crisis is precipitated by a hazardous event or a stressor, such as a catastrophe or disaster (e.g., earthquake, fire, war, terrorism), a relationship rupture or loss, sexual assault, or abuse. A crisis may also result from a series of difficult events or mishaps rather than from one major occurrence, and a crisis can be a response to external and internal stress. During crises, individuals perceive their lives, needs, security, relationships, and sense of well-being to be at risk. Crises tend to be time limited, generally lasting no more than a few months; the duration depends on the stressor and on the individual's perception of and response to the stressor.

Crisis states can lead to personal growth rather than physical and psychological deterioration (Caplan 1961). Crisis makes growth possible because it assaults the individual's psychic structure and defenses, throwing them into a state of flux, which can make the resilient individual more open to treatment. Davanloo (1980) incorporated production of a crisis into his short-term dynamic psychotherapy approach, viewing crisis as a means of disrupting ingrained defenses in order for patients to gain access to their inner lives and thereby change maladaptive ways of feeling, thinking, and behaving.

Crisis intervention is a therapeutic process aimed at restoring homeostatic balance and diminishing vulnerability to the stressor. The therapist helps the individual to accomplish homeostasis by mobilizing the individual's abilities and social network and promoting adaptive coping mechanisms to reestablish equilibrium. Crisis intervention is a short-term approach that focuses on solving the immediate problem and includes the entire therapeutic repertoire for helping patients deal with the challenges and threats of overwhelming stress.

An individual's reaction to stress is the result of a number of factors, including age, health, personality issues, prior experience with stressful events, emotional support, resources, belief systems, and underlying biological or genetic strengths or vulnerabilities. Traumatic events are common and varied and can be personal, such as the death of a loved one, sexual assault, the experience of being robbed, or involvement in a traffic accident. Other types of trauma, such as natural disasters or terrorist attacks, may involve large numbers of individuals, including persons not on the scene. The intensity and type of traumatic event is important, as is an individual's coping ability. At times, a series of traumatic events may produce a crisis that a single event would not have provoked. For example, a series of losses might result in a crisis that did not occur after the first few losses. Losses include death; separation; illness; financial loss; and loss of employment, function, or status.

The distinction between crisis intervention and psychotherapy is often blurred because the approaches may overlap in technique and length of treatment. Crisis intervention is generally expected to involve one to three contacts, whereas the duration of brief psychotherapy can extend from a few visits to 20 or more sessions. In this chapter, the term *crisis intervention* is also used for crisis-related treatment lasting longer than just a few sessions. This more inclusive form of crisis therapy is based on a number of different treatments, including dynamic supportive, cognitive-behavioral, humanistic, family, and systems approaches, as well as the use of medication when indicated. Systems approaches can be broad and can encompass actions such as working with and referral to social service agencies, clergy, mobile crisis units, suicide hotlines, and law enforcement agencies. In recent years, the focus of crisis intervention has been on emergency management and prevention through the use of various forms of debriefing.

Evaluation

According to Caplan (1961), ego assessment is key in the evaluation of an individual in a crisis situation. The evaluation consists of 1) examining the individual's capacity to deal with stress, maintain ego structure and equilibrium, and deal with reality, and 2) assessing problem-solving and coping abilities.

The evaluation of an individual in a crisis situation should be thorough and systematic but should also essentially be completed within the first session. A timely evaluation is critical because it enables the therapist to develop a case formulation and treatment plan and initiate treatment immediately. Even the evaluation session itself should be therapeutic to assist the patient in crisis. The evaluation should follow the process outlined in Chapter 3, "Assessment, Case Formulation, and Goal Setting," but also should focus on the traumatic situation, the precipitating event, and any possible danger the patient might pose to himself or herself or to others. The individual's experience of the trauma, including perceptions and feelings, and whether the person was a victim of or a witness to the traumatic event is important. The therapist should assess 1) the individual's current affect, anxiety level, and sense of hopefulness and 2) the way in which he or she attempts to deal with the trauma.

The following vignette illustrates the evaluation process in a broad-based, supportive psychotherapy–crisis intervention approach (see Video Vignette 5, Session 1, available at www.appi.org/Winston). The vignette includes excerpts from four sessions that began 6 months following the 2001 World Trade Center attack.

Video Vignette 5: Crisis Intervention

Session 1

William is a 44-year-old police officer with anxiety, depressive feelings, an inability to work, and difficulty enjoying anything about his life. He is tall, muscular, and physically imposing. In his first session, William reveals that he recently had a traumatic experience.

THERAPIST: So what's troubling you?

WILLIAM: I've just been having all kinds of problems in my life. I can't work; I can't sleep; I just don't enjoy anything anymore **(responds with multiple complaints)**.

THERAPIST: So you're having trouble working and sleeping, and you're not finding any enjoyment in your life. How long have you been having these difficulties? **(summarizes and attempts to find out when the patient's difficulties began)**

WILLIAM: It's been going on for about 6 months, but it's gotten worse over the last couple of months, I'd say.

THERAPIST: I see that your problems began 6 months ago. What was happening at that time? **(begins to focus on the beginning of the episode of illness)**

WILLIAM: Well, 9/11 happened. I was sent down there right at the beginning with three other policemen. It was terrible. I still can't believe what happened **(begins to talk about the traumatic events that occurred on September 11, 2001)**.

THERAPIST: Well, you know it is important that we try to go into as much detail as we can **(attempts to get details of the traumatic event and its effect on the patient)**. I know it might be difficult for you, but can you tell me what happened when you were at the World Trade Center? **(empathic)**

WILLIAM: We got down there. I was told to wait outside, and the other guys went in. They never came out.... I should have been there with them [*begins to cry*] **(is filled with emotion and perhaps feelings of guilt)**.

THERAPIST: I can see that this is very difficult for you **(responds in an empathic manner)**.

WILLIAM: Yeah. I was told to stay outside and monitor traffic, to make sure that no civilians got into the buildings.

THERAPIST: So you were outside, and they went in...and then what happened?

WILLIAM: Well, I was standing there just looking up, and I was stunned.... I saw people jumping.

THERAPIST: Oh my God! That must have been so frightening *(responds with emotion and in an empathic manner)*.

WILLIAM: Yeah…I saw a man and a woman…. They were holding hands…. They were jumping [*begins to sob*] *(gives further information)*.

THERAPIST: I'm so sorry you went through such a terrible ordeal. What a horror! I'm very, very sorry *(responds with emotion and in an empathic manner)*.

WILLIAM: That was only the first part of it. Then all of a sudden, the buildings began to shake and then—I couldn't believe it—one building started to come down, and I was buried. And all of a sudden, I looked up, and I saw my wife and my son holding hands and smiling and waving at me…. I thought I was dead.

THERAPIST: So you were buried, and you saw your wife and your son. You thought you were dead. How did you get through that experience? *(responds with a clarification, tracking, and admiration, and continues exploring)*

WILLIAM: At first I was completely paralyzed. I couldn't reason. My mind was totally confused. I felt like a mummy. I didn't move right away.

THERAPIST: And then what happened?

WILLIAM: I reached for my eyes, and I started to pull the stuff out of my eyes and out of my ears, and I stood up and I realized I was actually alive. I don't know how I got out. I saw a woman, and she was on her knees, and she had blood coming out of her forehead. I picked her up, and I took her to a rescue area. Then I went back in and found another man, and I carried him out also. *(Despite his horrendous ordeal, the patient behaved in a heroic manner.)*

THERAPIST: So you helped rescue two people! After everything you'd gone through, you rescued two people! *(praises and expresses admiration for his heroic behavior)*

WILLIAM: Yes, but I…the guys I came with…they never got out. I should have been there with them. I keep thinking about it. *(Despite his heroic behavior and the therapist's praise and admiration, the patient indicates that he feels guilty about not going in with the other policemen.)*

THERAPIST: You were a hero—and yet you still believe that you should have been there with them. Losing three fellow officers must have been very devastating for you *(praises the patient and begins to address the issue of his surviving while his fellow officers all died)*.

This vignette illustrates part of the process of evaluating a patient who is in a crisis situation and has a traumatic stress disorder. In the remainder of the evaluation, the therapist explores William's guilt about staying behind while others went in, his level of anxiety, and the extent of his depression. William's current family situation is examined, as well as his history. The following information emerges.

> William has been extremely anxious and tearful following his traumatic experience. He has been pacing back and forth in his home and thinking constantly about what happened to him on September 11, 2001. He has startle reactions to loud noises and has flashbacks about the building collapsing, people jumping, and seeing his wife and son. William has nightmares and thus avoids sleep. He can no longer concentrate, has little energy, feels helpless, and no longer enjoys anything in his life. He has been unable to return to work and tries to avoid anything that might remind him of September 11. His previous performance at work was quite good, and he was decorated on several occasions for heroism.
>
> William grew up in a middle-class family and had a good relationship with his mother. When he was 15 years old, his father died. William's relationship with his father had been difficult and filled with conflict, which resulted in mixed feelings toward his father. These feelings did not resolve when his father was dying, and they may have played a role in William's emphasis on bodybuilding and on presenting a strong manly image.

The therapist concludes that William has posttraumatic stress disorder (PTSD). Before the trauma, William was functioning at a high level and had good coping skills despite unresolved problems with his father. At present, his coping skills are no longer adequate, but he has a supportive spouse and appears to be motivated for psychotherapy. The treatment goals, formulated with William, include amelioration of his symptoms and a return to work. The treatment plan includes development of a supportive, positive therapeutic relationship at the onset of treatment, followed by work on symptom reduction with the use of exposure therapy, along with cognitive restructuring. Medication for anxiety and depression, such as a selective serotonin reuptake inhibitor, may also be indicated. As treatment progresses, a major focus will be to help William return to work as soon as possible.

Treatment

The therapeutic approaches used in crisis intervention are primarily those of brief supportive psychotherapy, consisting of maintenance of focus and a high therapist activity level; use of clearly established goals, a time limit, and a number of supportive and cognitive-behavioral interventions; and, most importantly, establishment of a solid therapeutic alliance. A number of systematic approaches to crisis intervention have been described (James and Gilliland 2001; Puryear 1979; Roberts 2000).

Systematic approaches to crisis intervention include stress assessment, patient safety, establishment of rapport and hopefulness, supportive interventions, and positive actions and plans. The importance of assessment was discussed in the previous section, "Evaluation." Patient safety is part of the assessment process and should be monitored throughout therapy if the individual's safety is in question (see the section "Suicide" later in this chapter). Establishing rapport and promoting hopefulness are important in all forms of psychotherapy and are major factors in fostering the therapeutic alliance. The major elements of the alliance (Gaston 1990) are the patient's affective bond with the therapist, the patient's ability to work purposefully and collaboratively with the therapist, the therapist's empathic understanding and involvement, and the agreement of patient and therapist on the goals and tasks of therapy. The use of supportive or empathic interventions helps promote the alliance, making it possible to use exposure techniques to help work through the patient's reaction to trauma. Positive actions and plans provide the patient with structure and improve self-esteem and hope for the future. Video Vignette 5 continues with sessions 2, 4, and 5 with William, the police officer with PTSD resulting from the events of September 11, 2001. These sessions illustrate the treatment process in a broad-based supportive psychotherapy crisis intervention approach.

 Video Vignette 5: Crisis Intervention *(continued)*

Session 2

William has completed his first session of supportive psychotherapy crisis intervention. In addition, treatment with a selective serotonin reuptake inhibitor has been started, with the dose gradually being increased to a therapeutic level during the course of treatment. The next two sessions are primarily directed at forming a secure and positive therapeutic alliance through the use of supportive interventions. Part of William's second session follows.

> WILLIAM: My wife told me that I don't bother with her anymore, that I just ignore her—but I don't feel like talking about anything,

doing anything.... I just don't feel like talking **(begins with a complaint from his wife rather than continuing to discuss the traumatic event—possibly a defensive move)**.

THERAPIST: You know last week at our first meeting, we explored what happened to you on that terrible day of 9/11, and something about your past life, and a bit concerning your relationship with your wife and son, and maybe today we can go into your current relationship with Cathy more in-depth **(chooses to address the patient's current issue with his wife to build a therapeutic relationship before going back to the traumatic event, which he may not be ready for at the current time; presents agenda)**.

WILLIAM: Well, Cathy comes over to me and tries to talk to me, to get me started talking, but I don't feel like talking; it's still too difficult **(indicates that he is overwhelmed, which may have implications for his feelings about talking to the therapist)**.

THERAPIST: OK. So it's really hard for you to talk, and I understand this. But perhaps there are some things that would be easier for you to talk about **(responds in an empathic manner and asks the patient to focus on areas that are less painful, anxiety provoking, and conflictual)**.

WILLIAM: It is really hard to talk about 9/11.... I like to talk about my son. I guess some things around the house. I like to do some gardening.

THERAPIST: So you could talk to Cathy about those things—about the house, your son, and so forth. Can you give me an example of what you might feel comfortable talking with Cathy about? **(always look for concrete examples)**

The therapist has recognized that William is having difficulty talking at home and is possibly having difficulty talking with the therapist. However, because William is talking spontaneously, the therapist has decided not to address the therapeutic relationship and instead has begun to focus on concrete areas that William can discuss with his wife. Focusing on concrete areas helps to reduce anxiety, which is important in both supportive psychotherapy and crisis intervention.

WILLIAM: Cathy wants Billy to go to sleep-away camp. I don't know—he's not much of an athlete, but he does like to play the saxophone. I kind of think it would be better if he just stayed home **(indicates his wish to have his son at home with him)**.

THERAPIST: Could it be that you disagree with Cathy because you would really like Billy to stay home with you? **(clarification, expressed tentatively)**

WILLIAM: I do like having him around **(ignores his conflict with his wife and focuses on his son)**.

THERAPIST: Yeah. So maybe I would be correct in saying that you want Billy to be with you, but you find it difficult to speak to Cathy about this directly? *(using a supportive approach, brings the patient back to his conflict with his wife; requests feedback)*

WILLIAM: That makes sense. I just can't be clear about what it is that I want, because I just really don't know *(agrees but indicates that he becomes passive and indecisive with his wife)*.

THERAPIST: It sounds like you would like to have Billy home this summer, but it's hard for you to be direct with Cathy, so you hang back and yet get annoyed with her. Is this correct? Do you agree with that? *(interprets the patient's wish to have his son home and his defensive posture of passivity and distraction accompanied by annoyance with his wife; again employs the supportive technique of asking for feedback so that the patient is not overwhelmed)*

The therapist has asked for a specific example of William's difficulty in communicating with his wife. Obtaining specific concrete examples from patients is always preferable to leaving things on a general level. When patients generalize, it is difficult to understand what they have in mind. In addition, it is not helpful to patients to remain in a confused or unclear state.

Having understood that William wishes to have his son at home, the therapist has been able to clarify this wish with William. The therapist has used a number of supportive approaches. Instead of addressing the transference, the therapist has continued to concentrate on William's current life and his difficulty with his wife, Cathy. In supportive psychotherapy, the transference generally is not addressed unless it is negative. Instead, the therapist concentrates on current issues in the patient's life and on the real relationship with the therapist. Clarification is used as a supportive technique because it does not place demands or expectations on the patient. In addition, the therapist has been able to link William's avoidance and annoyance with Cathy to his wish to keep Billy home for the summer and not have him go off to camp as Cathy wishes.

The pursuit of affect is generally avoided in supportive psychotherapy and has been avoided in this session. However, William's emotional experiences resulting from the World Trade Center tragedy will need to be addressed when exposure techniques are used later in therapy.

The therapist has determined that a good therapeutic relationship was established during the first three sessions (session 3 is not shown). Therefore, exposure therapy within a supportive framework can now be attempted to enable the patient to work through his traumatic experience, as shown in the following sessions 4 and 5.

Session 4

THERAPIST: William, I thought that we might go back and explore what happened to you on 9/11. If we can look at your experience together, it should help you to better deal with it and move on with your life. How do you feel about doing that now? *(The therapist asks for the patient's agreement to explore his traumatic experience. Asking for agreement constitutes the supportive technique of agenda setting.)*

WILLIAM: If it can help. I think I'm more ready.

THERAPIST: It's good that you feel ready and that we're able to proceed. Let's go back to that day when you went to the World Trade Center. OK? *(praises the patient and continues to involve him as a partner in planning the discussion)*

WILLIAM: OK.

THERAPIST: You and your fellow officers were sent to the World Trade Center about when? *(begins a detailed exploration of the patient's traumatic experience)*

WILLIAM: In the morning, after the second plane hit, we drove up.

Therapist: And as you were driving up, what were you experiencing?

WILLIAM: The fires were just raging. We knew by then that it was an attack. We met the sergeant, and he told me I should stay outside to keep people out, as I said before.

THERAPIST: What was it like for you, remaining outside while the others went in? *(is aware of the patient's not wanting to remain behind and his guilt feelings about being the only survivor from his group)*

WILLIAM: I wanted to go in with them.

THERAPIST: So how did you feel? *(For the first time the therapist asks about the patient's feelings. Exposure therapy relies on the patient's experiencing and exploring feelings, in a somewhat controlled fashion, during the session.)*

WILLIAM: Standing around, I felt useless. I was annoyed. I didn't want to stay behind.

THERAPIST: That's understandable, but you were ordered to stay behind *(absolution as a supportive technique)*.

The therapist has emphasized that William was ordered to stay behind because during the evaluation session, William indicated that he felt guilty and conflicted about staying outside. The therapist is preparing the groundwork for addressing William's cognitive distortion of this issue and his possible survivor guilt.

The session continues with a recounting of the traumatic events that followed.

WILLIAM: I was standing there in the street. Then all of a sudden, I saw people jumping from the building. Some of them were on fire.
THERAPIST: That's horrible! What were you feeling? *(asks William for his feelings in an empathic manner to promote exploration and desensitization)*
WILLIAM: It was hard to look...[*begins to sob*]. I couldn't believe it. Then I saw a man and a woman jumping, and they were holding hands! [*becomes visibly shaken and anxious*]
THERAPIST: Who wouldn't be devastated, shaken, and tearful? *(clarifies in an empathic manner using the supportive technique of normalizing)*

The therapist has been obtaining a detailed account of William's traumatic experience and has also been monitoring his level of anxiety to ensure that it remains within manageable limits. If a patient's anxiety level gets too high, the therapist can slow down the account and initiate anxiety-lowering interventions, such as having the patient engage in progressive muscular relaxation and deep breathing or meditation. In addition to these techniques, which are generally used in exposure therapy, supportive interventions such as reassurance can also be used.

The session continues with a detailed exploration of William's experiences of that day, including the collapse of the buildings, his near burial in the debris, his hallucination of his wife and son, and his belief that he was dead. The therapist elicits these experiences in great detail and in an empathic manner, with careful monitoring of William's anxiety level. During the exploration of William's vision of his wife and son—the vision in which he saw them holding hands and waving good-bye to him—William becomes visibly shaken and anxious because at that time he believed he was dead. The therapist stops the exploration and begins anxiety-lowering techniques of meditation with deep breathing and the use of a mantra.

Session 5

Session 5 begins with a discussion of the patient's anxiety level during the interval between sessions. This information is important because the aim in supportive therapy is to keep anxiety level as low as possible. William indicates that he has not been experiencing a significant amount of anxiety between sessions.

THERAPIST: Do you think you feel ready now to continue exploring what happened to you on that day on 9/11? *(checks to see if*

> *the patient is ready to continue exposure therapy; again*
> *uses the supportive technique of agenda setting)*

WILLIAM: Yeah…I can keep going.

THERAPIST: You're very strong, and you have a lot of resilience. So, let's pick up where we left off: after you saw your wife and son. Is that OK? *(offers praise—a supportive intervention—and then resumes exploration of the patient's traumatic experience)*

WILLIAM: Yeah, I began to realize that I wasn't actually dead, and I started to push away all the stuff off me…out of my face, ears, and eyes. It was all over me *(continues without much difficulty)*.

THERAPIST: So as you began to realize you were not dead, how did you feel?

WILLIAM: I certainly felt some relief…. I thought, thank God—thank God, I'm all right. Then I got up and I saw a woman on her knees. She was bleeding from her scalp, blood was coming down her face. All I thought to do was help her up and carry her out to the rescue area.

THERAPIST: Yeah. So despite your being battered and even thinking you were dead just a few minutes earlier, you were still able to pull a woman out of the rubble and rescue her. That's amazing! *(offers praise and expresses admiration—both useful supportive interventions, provided that the praise and admiration are clearly reality based and deserved)*

The therapist goes on to explore the details of William's next few hours after he picked himself up from the rubble. These details include rescuing a man, going to the hospital to have lacerations sutured, and finding out that the three policemen who went into the building had died. All these experiences are fully explored during the next few sessions, until William can talk about his experience without too much anxiety or overwhelming sadness.

William's treatment involves the use of exposure therapy in the context of a supportive relationship. The therapist is able to take William through his traumatic experience in a slow and detailed manner over the course of several meetings. The therapist monitors William's anxiety level so that he is not overwhelmed. If William begins to become overly aroused, the therapist stops the exposure work and uses a number of supportive techniques, such as praise, reassurance, and relaxation therapy along with meditation. At the same time, a great deal of work is required to restructure William's excessive feelings of guilt about being the only survivor of his group of four policemen. The therapist challenges William's self-blaming cognitions to help him reframe his idea that he should have been inside the World Trade Center with his fellow officers (cognitive restructuring). The therapist points out that William was ordered to remain outside the building and helps him understand the concept of survivor guilt when she states, "Many people who survive tragedies as you did feel guilty."

After 10 sessions, William gradually improves and is able to return to work and to feel comfortable with his wife and son. He still has episodes of anxiety and sadness, which he is able to manage, and he continues taking medication. He has two follow-up sessions, 1 month later and then 3 months later, to prevent relapse.

Treatment Approaches for PTSD

In this chapter we have described the treatment of PTSD using supportive psychotherapy combined with exposure therapy and cognitive restructuring, along with the anxiety-reducing techniques of progressive muscular relaxation and meditation. A number of other treatment approaches have been used in PTSD with good results. These include cognitive therapy (Foa et al. 2005); eye movement desensitization and reprocessing (van der Kolk et al. 2007); interpersonal therapy (Markowitz et al. 2015); mantram repetition (Bormann et al. 2018); and the use of virtual reality for patients with treatment-resistant PTSD, especially military veterans (van Gelderen et al. 2018). Cusack et al. (2016) completed a systematic review and meta-analysis assessing the efficacy and comparative effectiveness of a number of these therapies and found that exposure therapy had the greatest strength of evidence for effectiveness. Unfortunately, most psychotherapy approaches do not combine different treatments to form an integrated psychotherapy. The treatment of William's PTSD used an integrated psychotherapy approach combining supportive psychotherapy, exposure treatment, cognitive restructuring, and anxiety-reducing techniques. Supportive psychotherapy easily lends itself to an integrated, multifaceted psychotherapy.

Suicide

The prediction of suicide is problematic because there is no reliable way of determining suicidal risk in a given individual within a given time frame (Chiles et al. 2019; Fawcett et al. 1993; Pokorny 1983). Two major problems occur when attempts are made to predict suicide: 1) too many false-positive cases are identified and 2) many instances of completed suicide are overlooked. Nevertheless, more than 90% of completed suicides occur in individuals with a recent major psychiatric illness (Fawcett et al. 1993). The most common diagnoses are major depression, chronic alcoholism and drug abuse, schizophrenia, borderline personality disorder, bipolar disorder, and eating disorders. Retrospective case review studies of completed suicides suggest heightened suicide risk in the context of a recent traumatic loss, such as a breakup in an important relationship, being fired from a job, or losing status or a place of belonging (Joiner 2005). A careful and thorough assessment of the suicidal patient is critical to determine the diagnosis and the proper treatment approach. Crisis intervention approaches, generally accompanied by the use of medication, often play an important role in the treatment of suicidal individuals.

Assessment of Risk

Suicidal thoughts and behaviors are so common that it is essential to ask all patients about suicidal ideas and attempts. A history of suicide attempts increases a person's risk for completing suicide. Individuals who have well-defined plans to kill themselves are at greater risk than individuals with vague or poorly formulated plans. When a suicidal person has the means to end his or her life and has great familiarity with the means (e.g., owns and uses a firearm), the patient is at greater and often significant risk. The presence of strong family support or a significant other can have a mitigating effect on suicidal risk. Hopelessness, pessimism, aggression, impulsiveness, and psychic anxiety are poor prognostic signs. Another factor to be considered, as noted earlier, is the loss of a significant other through separation, divorce, or death.

Paradoxically, it was found that more than half of patients who died by suicide had consulted clinicians within 1 year before death and had denied suicidal thoughts or indicated that they rarely occurred (Clark and Fawcett 1992). Often, these same patients communicated directly or indirectly to a close friend or relative that they were thinking of ending their lives. This information suggests that physicians should routinely question close relatives and friends of patients who may be at risk for suicide.

Fawcett et al. (1990, 1993) divided suicidal risk into acute and chronic categories. Individuals who are at acute risk often have severe anxiety, thoughts about negative events occurring, insomnia, anhedonia, agitation, and alcohol abuse (Busch et al. 2003). Persons at more chronic risk have more typical risk factors, such as suicidal ideation and plans and a history of suicide attempts.

The risk of suicide is often greatest during the week after hospital admission and the month after discharge and during the early period of recovery from a psychiatric disorder (Hawton 1987). For a comprehensive review and discussion of imminent suicide risk, see the book *The Suicidal Crisis: A Clinical Guide to the Assessment of Imminent Suicide Risk* by Igor Galynker (2017).

Treatment

Suicidal thoughts represent a form of problem-solving by patients in tremendous and unrelenting psychological pain. Acknowledging the patient's pain, helping him or her to find ways to reduce the burden of pain, and assisting the patient in identifying alternative solutions to suicide are important tasks in establishing a therapeutic alliance and implementing treatment during the suicidal crisis (Chiles et al. 2019). The therapist should explore the patient's perspective and life story along several considerations: the patient's belief in suicide as a solution to a particular problem; the patient's past history of suicidal behavior and its impact on others; the patient's ability to tolerate significant pain; the patient's reasons for *not* committing suicide, should this be possible; and the patient's perceptions of a future that *could* be positive (Chiles et al. 2019).

Therapists, especially those who are very sensitive to the inner experiences of their patients and those who are early in their training or clinical practice, may feel overwhelmed by the suffering felt and expressed by suicidal patients. To be effective in working in crisis settings with suicidal patients, it is very important that therapists recognize their own feelings and ensure that they are able to respond in an open and constructive manner that creates physical and emotional safety for the patient.

Once an individual has been determined to be acutely suicidal, hospitalization may be indicated. If hospitalization is not feasible or not absolutely necessary, the therapist should enlist the aid of significant others who can spend time with the patient and not leave the patient alone. The therapist needs to be available for contact either by the patient or by the patient's family or friends and should provide them with information regarding 24-hour hotlines and the nearest emergency department. Medication is often necessary in the short term to relieve the patient's anxiety, agitation, or depression. The frequency of treatment sessions will vary depending on the patient's needs. Some patients may need to be seen daily for ongoing support and structure. Accordingly, it is important that the same clinician see the patient throughout the period of crisis intervention. Important issues on which to focus are patient hopelessness and pessimism. Supportive approaches involving praise, reassurance, and cognitive restructuring are often useful to help enhance self-esteem by counteracting negative or distorted cognitions about the self. As always, establishment and maintenance of a positive therapeutic alliance are essential.

Crisis Intervention Versus Psychotherapy

As stated in the section "History and Theory" at the beginning of this chapter, crisis intervention theory is based on a number of psychological approaches, including dynamic supportive psychotherapy, cognitive-behavioral therapy, humanistic treatments, family therapy, and systems approaches. Crisis intervention is time limited and is not focused on psychological insight, personality issues, or psychiatric disorders. An individual receiving crisis intervention is generally in transition or has lost his or her equilibrium because of a traumatic experience that has disrupted his or her life. Patients vary in their resilience and sources of support. The objective of crisis intervention is to help the individual deal with the stressful period, achieve stability, and return to his or her precrisis level of functioning or, if the patient needs further treatment, move on to the next level of care.

Crisis intervention differs from psychotherapy in a number of ways (outlined in Table 7–1). Crisis treatment is given as soon as possible and in close proximity to the stressor or traumatic event. It is time limited, and the therapist is active, supportive, and directive. As in supportive psychotherapy (as opposed to expressive psychotherapy), the focus is on the here and now rather than on the past or on transference issues.

Critical Incident Stress Management

Critical incident stress management (CISM) was originally developed for use with emergency workers; however, its scope has been expanded to include anyone exposed to severe trauma (Everly and Mitchell 1999; Mitchell and Everly 2003). CISM is a comprehensive and integrated crisis intervention approach for individuals and groups. The components of CISM are summarized in Table 7–2 and include the following: precrisis preparation involving stress management education and training for individuals and groups of professional and emergency workers; briefings on disasters and terrorist or other large-scale incidents for rescue workers and civilians; defusing (i.e., immediate small-group discussion) to ensure assessment and triage and to mitigate symptoms; critical incident stress debriefing (CISD; Mitchell and Everly 1996) to reduce impairments from traumatic stress, facilitate closure, and mitigate symptoms for individuals and groups; individual or family crisis intervention; and follow-up and referral for further assessment and treatment.

A typical CISD approach after a traumatic event involves a group of victims who undergo the interventions, listed in Table 7–2, in a single 1- to 3-hour session. The efficacy of a single-session debriefing in preventing PTSD or other disorders came into question in 2002. In a meta-analysis of single-session debriefing within 1 month after trauma, van Emmerik et al. (2002) found that CISD interventions do not improve natural recovery from psychological trauma. However, single-session approaches of this sort may help reduce immediate distress and facilitate referral of patients for

Table 7–1. Crisis intervention versus psychotherapy

	Crisis intervention	Psychotherapy
Context	Prevention	Reparation
Timing	Immediate; close temporal relationship to stressor or acute decompensation	Delayed; distant from stressor or acute decompensation
Location	Close proximity to stressor or acute decompensation; anywhere needed	Safe, secure environment
Duration	Typically one to three contacts	As long as needed or desired
Provider's role	Active, directive	Guiding, collaborative, consultative
Strategic foci	Conscious processes, environmental stressors or factors	Conscious and unconscious sources of pathogenesis
Temporal focus	Here and now	Present and past
Patient expectations	Symptom reduction, reduction of impairment, directive support	Symptom reduction, reduction of impairment, personal growth, guidance, collaboration
Goals	Stabilization, reduction of impairment, a return to function or a shift to next level of care	Symptom reduction, reduction of impairment, correction of pathogenesis, personal growth, personal reconstruction

Source. Aguilera et al. 1970; Artiss 1963; Everly and Mitchell 1998; Koss and Shiang 1994; Salmon 1919; Sandoval 1985; Skaikeu 1990; Spiegel and Classen 1995; Wilkinson and Vera 1985.
Reprinted from Everly GS Jr, Mitchell JT: *Critical Incident Stress Management (CISM): A New Era and Standard of Care in Crisis Intervention,* 2nd Edition. Ellicott City, MD, Chevron Publishing, 1999. Used with permission.

Table 7–2. Core components of critical incident stress management

Intervention	Timing	Activation	Goals	Recipients
Precrisis preparation	Precrisis	Driven by crisis anticipation	Setting of expectations, improved coping, stress management	Individuals, groups, organizations
Demobilization and staff consultation (rescuers)	Shift disengagement	Event driven	Presentation of information, consultation, psychological decompression, stress management	Organizations, large groups
Crisis management briefing (civilians, schools, businesses)	Anytime postcrisis	Event driven	Presentation of information, consultation, psychological decompression, stress management	Organizations, large groups
Defusing	Postcrisis (within 12 hours)	Usually symptom driven	Symptom mitigation, possible closure, triage	Small groups
Critical incident stress debriefing	Postcrisis (1–10 days; mass disasters: 3–4 weeks)	Usually symptom driven; sometimes event driven	Facilitation of psychological closure, symptom mitigation, triage	Individuals, small groups
Individual crisis intervention	Anytime, anywhere	Symptom driven	Symptom mitigation, possible return to function, referral if needed	Individuals
Family crisis intervention	Anytime	Symptom or event driven	Fostering of support and communication	Families

Table 7-2. Core components of critical incident stress management (*continued*)

Intervention	Timing	Activation	Goals	Recipients
Community and organizational consultation	Anytime	Symptom or event driven	Symptom mitigation, possible closure, referral if needed	Organizations
Pastoral crisis intervention	Anytime	Usually symptom driven	"Crisis of faith" mitigation, use of spiritual tools to assist in recovery	Individuals, families, groups
Follow-up and referral	Anytime	Usually symptom driven	Mental status assessment, a shift to higher level of care if needed	Individuals, families

Source. Adapted from Everly GS Jr, Mitchell JT: *Critical Incident Stress Management (CISM): A New Era and Standard of Care in Crisis Intervention,* 2nd Edition. Ellicott City, MD, Chevron Publishing, 1999. Used with permission.

further treatment. Positive outcomes have been achieved with cognitive-behavioral treatments that were administered within the first month of the traumatic incident and that involved education, exposure, and cognitive restructuring (Bryant et al. 1999; Foa 1997; Foa et al. 1991).

Conclusion

In this chapter, we provided a brief history and the theoretical background of crisis intervention. Individuals exposed to severe trauma can react in a number of ways, and some of these reactions necessitate crisis intervention. A thorough evaluation of a patient presenting in crisis is always necessary. Treatment approaches vary depending on the needs of the patient but generally include supportive interventions, exposure therapy, cognitive restructuring, and anxiety-reducing techniques. A patient's suicidal thoughts represent a form of problem-solving—a way of escaping tremendous and unrelenting psychological pain. Therapists must pay particular attention to establishing and maintaining a positive therapeutic alliance. Acknowledging and lessening the patient's pain and finding alternative solutions to suicide are important tasks in establishing a therapeutic alliance and implementing treatment during a suicidal crisis. The terrorist attacks of September 11, 2001, in New York and Washington, D.C.; the 2010 Haiti earthquake; and the increased number of terrorist attacks, tornadoes, hurricanes, and floods in recent years, as well as battlefield injuries, have made both the general public and mental health professionals more aware of these issues and the need for crisis intervention services.

Applicability to Special Populations

8

Severe Mental Illness

As originally conceived, supportive psychotherapy was indicated for patients with severe mental illness, as well as for other patients for whom expressive treatment was not indicated. The original indication for supportive psychotherapy was treatment at the extreme supportive end of the supportive-expressive psychotherapy continuum described in Chapter 1, "Evolution of the Concept of Supportive Psychotherapy." This form of supportive treatment was focused primarily on improving deficient ego functions, reducing anxiety, and preventing downward social drift due to loss of adaptive skills and increasing isolation. In addition to offering the patient an understanding, supportive relationship, this approach contained many of the following techniques: advice, reassurance, exhortation, praise, encouragement, lending ego, and environmental manipulation. Supporting defenses was the default mode, confrontation was rare, and interpretation did not occur.

In current practice, even for patients who are quite impaired because of severe mental illness, therapists should strive for a balance between supportive and expressive elements in supportive treatment. Depending on several factors—including the degree of stabilization after acute exacerbation of illness, the strength of the therapeutic alliance (see Chapter 6, "The Therapeutic Relationship"), and the patient's treatment goals—confrontation and, at times, interpretation can be useful techniques in supportive psychotherapy. Cognitive learning strategies, such as teaching, using slogans, modeling, and giving anticipatory guidance, are commonly used. The treatment components of psychoeducation and skills training, which have been framed as independent interventions, are consistent with the model of supportive treatment and are particularly useful in supportive psychotherapy for chronic mental illness.

Schizophrenia

Schizophrenia is the prototypical severe mental illness. When treating a patient who has schizophrenia, the therapist provides education about the illness, promotes medication compliance, facilitates reality testing, encourages problem solving by the patient, and reinforces adaptive behavior with praise (Lamberti and Herz 1995). Gunderson et al. (1984) demonstrated that patients with schizophrenia have better treatment retention and better outcome when given weekly supportive treatment rather than more intensive expressive treatment.

Praise is a form of reinforcement that can support the patient's self-esteem and motivation for adaptive change. As described in detail in Chapter 4, "Techniques," praise is an important esteem-building technique. However, praise builds self-esteem only when the praised behavior is considered praiseworthy by the patient. Therefore, the therapist must understand what the patient will find worthy of praise. The therapist also must attempt to understand what the patient finds rewarding so that these incentives can be enlisted to provide positive feedback. Determining what the patient finds rewarding is especially important in schizophrenia and at the left side of the psychopathology continuum, where positive reinforcement is an important factor in maintaining the therapeutic alliance and motivating engagement in treatment.

Positive reinforcement is helpful for patients with schizophrenia because they commonly have neurocognitive impairments; negative symptoms, such as apathy, anhedonia, and poor motivation; and poor insight. A reinforcer can be a favorite food, activity, person, or social event that increases the strength or frequency of the patient's contingent behavior. Properly assessed and delivered reinforcers increase patients' skill acquisition, achievement of goals, and self-esteem (Lecomte et al. 2000). External rewards that patients value may be helpful in engaging and maintaining these patients in treatment. Rewards can include subway tokens, certificates of accomplishment, a celebratory event, and gift certificates. Administration of accurate praise, as described throughout this book, is an effective and inexpensive reward.

Psychoeducation

Typically, supportive psychotherapy for patients with severe mental illness includes psychoeducation about the illness, its trajectory, and its treatment. The literature suggests that educating patients about schizophrenia or substance dependence reinforces psychosocial rehabilitation (Goldman and Quinn 1988). Most patients generally find learning new information to be supportive. When provided in an empathic way, psychoeducation offers the patient a new cognitive structure on which to base more realistic decision making. Psychoeducation also gives the patient an explanation of or rationale for symptoms and suffering; giving such explanations or rationales may also bolster the patient's self-esteem.

In addition, concrete information about the illness arms the patient with practical knowledge that can help improve his or her ability to cope with chronic illness—an adaptive skill. For example, early in an exacerbation of the manic phase of bipolar disorder, the patient frequently loses the capacity to understand that his or her judgment is impaired by mania. During a remission, the psychiatrist can teach the patient that sleeping even 1 hour less than usual for 2 nights in a row may be an early sign of relapse into mania. This information gives the patient an opportunity to demonstrate some adaptive mastery over the illness and to act before an exacerbation can impair judgment and destroy the chance to "step on the brakes." For example, when the symptom of impaired sleep occurs and the patient contacts the psychiatrist for a dose escalation of antimanic medication, the patient will likely experience increased self-efficacy and self-esteem. These positive effects will occur as a result of the patient's sense of increased competence in anticipating potentially damaging future events and will strengthen the therapeutic alliance.

Supporting Adaptive Skills

To help patients who have impairments in interpersonal functioning secondary to severe mental disorders such as schizophrenia, the therapist can integrate behavioral skills training and other cognitive-behavioral techniques into supportive psychotherapy. The model of change in supportive therapy is change through learning and through introjection of or identification with an accepting, well-related therapist (Pinsker et al. 1991). Training in social and independent living skills for patients with severe mental illness is an approach grounded in learning principles, wherein the therapist breaks down complex social repertoires and models correct behavior for the patient, who repeatedly practices the skills after learning them. After the steps are assembled, the patient practices the complex interaction—first with the therapist, then in the real world. The therapist uses supportive techniques, such as behavioral goal setting, encouragement, modeling, shaping, and praise (positive reinforcement), to teach interpersonal skills (Glynn et al. 2002). This activity directly supports adaptive skills and builds patients' self-esteem. Studies have demonstrated the utility of these interventions in improving social competence (Heinssen et al. 2000; Lauriello et al. 1999).

Patients with schizophrenia have social skills deficits, which may be a result of impaired information processing. Skills training uses the problem-solving, repetitive, and practical approach of supportive psychotherapy and is effective in improving basic conversational skills, recreational skills, medication management, and management of symptoms (Liberman et al. 1998; Smith et al. 1999). A related cognitive-behavioral approach, relapse prevention, is discussed in the subsection "Adaptive Skills and Relapse Prevention" later in this chapter.

At times, the clinician must balance his or her focus on anxiety reduction as a major supportive strategy with the patient's determination to work through a particular problem, which could increase the patient's adaptive skills. For example, a patient might become anxious on hearing certain information about schizophrenia from the therapist. However, providing guidance about hearing the information and reframing the content in an attempt to strengthen the patient's coping skills may reduce the patient's anxiety. Having more extensive coping strategies that use higher-level defenses (e.g., rationalization) can mean that the patient has a more flexible and adaptive approach to his or her illness. At other times, when the patient signals that he or she is experiencing too much anxiety to deal with a subject directly, it can be useful for the therapist to attempt to "back into" discussion of the difficult topic.

THERAPIST: So, I would like to talk to you about what you understand about your illness. Is that OK with you? *("shows the map" before exploring the territory)*
PATIENT: I guess.
THERAPIST: If what I'm saying doesn't make sense to you, please tell me, and I'll try to clarify it. If it makes you more nervous, let me know, and we'll talk about something else. OK? *(offers anticipatory guidance about material to be explored, gives patient permission to stop the exploration, sets a collaborative tone, and indicates that the therapist is sensitive to the patient's feelings)*
PATIENT: All right.
THERAPIST: Has anyone discussed with you what your diagnosis is? That means the medical name of the illness that's bringing you into psychiatric treatment.
PATIENT: Uh, depression. I have depression.
THERAPIST: That's what they told you?

PATIENT: I don't know…um, I have depression.*(Patient has been told previously that his diagnosis is schizophrenia. He is either being evasive or using denial.)*

THERAPIST: Could you describe for me what the word *depression* means to you?

PATIENT: Yeah, I couldn't sleep, and I don't do much. Don't feel like it. I used to do things.

THERAPIST: Any other problems, like in your thoughts or feelings?

PATIENT: I have depression *(concrete, perseverative, nonelaborative answer)*.

THERAPIST: Are you sad a lot? People who are depressed are often sad.

PATIENT: No, not sad. I just don't feel much of anything. Tired. I don't know *(disclaims a low mood associated with depression)*.

THERAPIST: OK. Now, other than being tired, are there things you've been experiencing lately that have caused you problems?

PATIENT: Huh? Like what? [*suspicious look*]

THERAPIST: Well, you told the other doctor back in your intake evaluation that you had been thinking that somebody or maybe some group was trying to harm you, that you saw evidence of that. Is that accurate?

PATIENT: That was before. I don't think about it now [*looks away*] *(engages in distancing and avoiding)*.

THERAPIST: Can you tell me a little about what you were thinking and experiencing then? *(asks about patient's experience)*

PATIENT: Scary, uh…don't want to talk about it. I don't think about it now *(focusing on persecutory delusion increases patient's anxiety)*.

THERAPIST: OK, I won't ask you about the details. So, now it's not on your mind. You said it was before. Before when? I didn't understand what you meant *(moves away from past experience; asks for clarification of patient's statement)*.

PATIENT: You know, when I went on the pills for depression, it got better.

THERAPIST: Ah, so you don't have those scary thoughts so much since you started taking the medication? It's good you're taking it! *(clarifies, connecting medication and relief from delusional thinking; adds praise)*

PATIENT: Yeah. That's true.

THERAPIST: So, let me clarify: the medication you're taking seems to have a good impact on scary thoughts and experiences. Is that accurate?

PATIENT: That's true [*eye contact, brightens a little*].

THERAPIST: So I guess it's a good idea to keep taking it? *(ties what patient experiences as beneficial to a motivating statement for medication adherence)*

PATIENT: Yeah! And I talk to people better. They don't seem so negative to me *(validates therapist's position)*.

THERAPIST: So the medication helps you communicate better, too? Does that mean you get along with people better than before?

PATIENT: I keep to myself pretty much. But I don't get into fights like I did *(the patient is more elaborative as anxiety is reduced in situ)*.

THERAPIST: You mean you got into physical fights?

PATIENT: Only one time. Mostly just yelling back at some of the people when I knew what they were up to.

THERAPIST: What were they up to? *(asks for clarification)*

PATIENT: They were trying to make me look bad—said bad things about me from down the street [*looks away*]. Hmm, I don't think about it now *(starts to demonstrate increased anxiety, repeating his reflexive phrase)*.

THERAPIST: So that's better now, too? That's good. What else is better? *(goes along with the resistance; moves back to the present to reduce anxiety)*

PATIENT: My walls are quiet. I sleep better.

THERAPIST: How were they noisy?

PATIENT: The lady upstairs was making noise at night.

THERAPIST: What kind of noises? Like playing music too loud? Moving furniture?

PATIENT: No, uh, she would say ugly, ugly things to me. I couldn't sleep; I'd have to stay up.

THERAPIST: How would she talk to you?

PATIENT: I don't know—but it came from the wall.

THERAPIST: So you were hearing her voice telling you things you found unpleasant and you couldn't sleep? And it's better now? *(clarifies)*

PATIENT: Yes, I can sleep again.

THERAPIST: That must have been a terrible time for you. I'm glad you're feeling better. What a relief that must be! *(gives an empathic response based on patient's statements)*

PATIENT: Uh-huh [*smiles*].

THERAPIST: I'm going to summarize what you've told me the medication does for you, so we're clear I have it right. It takes away scary thoughts and experiences, takes away voices at night and helps you to sleep, and lets you get along with people better.

PATIENT: That's it.

THERAPIST: Sounds like good medicine!

PATIENT: It works.

THERAPIST: So can we get back to that illness that gave you the scary thoughts and experiences like voices, that kept you up, and that made it hard to get along with people? *(again "shows the map")*

PATIENT: OK.

THERAPIST: The medicine you are taking treats those symptoms of a disorder called schizophrenia—and, as we've just talked about, treats them pretty well: you're feeling a lot better than before.

PATIENT: I don't have that! My face didn't change. I don't attack people and drink their blood. My face didn't change *(becomes anxious and derails; reveals his delusional fears)*.

THERAPIST: I think maybe you're confusing an idea you have about vampires—that maybe you saw on TV—with schizophrenia. Vampires aren't real. Schizophrenia is, but it's a treatable mental disorder that has exactly the symptoms you've already described to me—symptoms that the medicine you take is good at controlling. You are not some kind of soulless monster *(reality tests, clarifies, confronts, and reassures)*.

PATIENT: What's going to happen to me? [*tears up*]

THERAPIST: We have better medicines and better therapies than ever before, and I will be here and work with you so that you can improve the quality of your life.

Family Psychoeducation

When supportive treatment is used with higher-functioning patients, environmental manipulation generally is not employed. With more impaired patients, however, the therapist can judiciously intervene in the patient's environment to support continued adaptation and reduce anxiety and stress. A clear example of this approach is family psychoeducation, in which educating the family changes the patient's environment. Teaching the family about the nature of the patient's disorder can help stabilize the family members around the patient in a way that is more supportive of the patient's recovery. Family stabilization is in contrast to the family making the patient the focus of their disappointment, failed expectations, criticism, disbelief, and ignorance. Such family reactions are unlikely to help a patient better cope with chronic illness; some family behaviors, such as high expressed emotion, are clearly associated with exacerbation of illness (Vaughn and Leff 1976). Indeed, short-term family intervention in families with high expressed emotion reduces relapse rates among patients with schizophrenia (Bellack and Mueser 1993).

Personality Disorders

For most therapists, the patients who are most difficult to treat are not the sickest patients (i.e., those with psychotic symptoms and profound impairment of ego functioning) but rather the patients who are highly angry, demanding, suspicious, or dependent (Horowitz and Marmar 1985). Patients with personality disorders use pervasive, maladaptive interpersonal strategies, and their behaviors are sometimes dangerous or frightening. Therefore, these patients can provoke strong negative emotions in people—including psychiatrists, who may avoid treating patients with personality disorders (Lewis and Appleby 1988). The treatability of this class of disorders is contingent on several factors, including disorder severity; the specific diagnosis; the patient's degree of involvement with medical, social, and criminal justice systems; comorbidity; the availability of appropriately trained staff; and the state of scientific knowledge (Adshead 2001).

Clearly, persons administering supportive treatment to such patients must have adequate training or supervision to deal with inevitable countertransference issues, as discussed in Chapter 6. Nonetheless, supportive psychotherapy is particularly suited to the treatment of most personality disorders because this therapy focuses on increasing self-esteem and adaptive skills while developing and maintaining a strong therapeutic alliance. As described in Chapter 3, "Assessment, Case Formulation, and Goal Setting," the psychiatrist must conduct an assessment of the patient that allows for a case formulation, including an explication of ego functioning, adaptive skills, object relations, and defensive operations.

In certain clusters of personality disorders, patients appear to make greater use of particular groups of maladaptive defenses and defensive behaviors. For example, in the treatment of patients with avoidant personality disorder, a major focus is on getting the patient to develop skills to overcome passivity and fears of rejection. In contrast, in the treatment of patients with narcissistic personality disorder, the focus is on addressing and reducing uses of externalization and criticism. The clinician decides at what point to use more containing, anxiety-reducing supportive technique and when to use more expressive technique. In particular, because clarification is the expressive technique used most frequently in supportive psychotherapy, within the supportive psychotherapy frame, clarification can elucidate maladaptive constructs that contribute to the patient's interpersonal problems and experienced loss of self-efficacy. Through implementation of techniques focused on adaptive skills, patients may develop a less rigid and more adaptive set of responses (Sachse and Kramer 2018).

Identifying comorbid mood and anxiety disorders is important in patients with personality disorders. In contrast to earlier concerns that medicating patients would deprive them of the motivation for engagement in treatment, today it is recognized that judicious pharmacological treatment of comorbid depression and anxiety disorders generally acts synergistically with the patients' attempts to learn and master new adaptive skills. In depressed patients, pharmacotherapy reduces Cluster C personality pathology—in particular, harm avoidance, which is associated with poor social function (Hellerstein et al. 2000; Kool et al. 2003; Peselow et al. 1994). When patients are less anxious or less depressed, they are more willing to explore new strategies and may be better able to do so (see Chapter 3 for an evaluation of a patient with major depressive disorder).

In a review of the effectiveness of psychotherapies for personality disorder, Perry et al. (1999) found that all studies of active psychotherapies reported positive outcomes at termination and follow-up. In addition, patients receiving treatment have an accelerated rate of recovery from personality disorders compared with the natural course of the disorders. Bateman and Fonagy (2000) conducted a systematic review of the evidence for efficacy of psychotherapy in personality disorders. Although psychotherapy was found to be effective, the evidence did not indicate that one form of treatment was superior to another. Effective treatments were found to have several factors in common, including encouragement of a strong patient-therapist relationship that would allow the therapist to take an active rather than passive stance.

Rosenthal et al. (1999) demonstrated lasting change in interpersonal functioning among patients with Cluster C personality disorders who were treated with 40 sessions of manual-based supportive psychotherapy. In patients with major depressive and personality disorders (especially Cluster C personality disorders), short-term (16-session) supportive psychotherapy in combination with antidepressant treatment led to greater reduction in personality pathology compared with antidepressant treatment alone (Kool et al. 2003). Patients with problems of hostile dominance, such as patients with antisocial personality disorder, tend to receive less demonstrable benefit from supportive psychotherapy than do patients with other personality disorders (Kool et al. 2003; Woody et al. 1985); however, when patients with antisocial personality disorder have comorbid depression, they may do well with supportive psychotherapy. Gerstley et al. (1989) hypothesized that the benefit is related to the patients' having some capacity to form a therapeutic alliance.

In supportive psychotherapy, it has been posited that when transference interpretation does not occur, the character-transforming factor may be the patient's capacity to form an identification with the more benign, accepting attitude of the therapist (Appelbaum and Levy 2002; Pinsker et al. 1991). For example, patients with borderline personality disorder typically must contend with what in structural terms is thought of as a rigid, archaic, and punitive superego. Identification with the therapist may allow the patient to be more tolerant of hateful and shameful aspects of the self.

Holmes (1995) reported on borderline patients' use of the commitment, concern, and attention to the supportive technique during psychoanalytic treatment and suggested that the development of secure attachments fostered more autonomous functioning. By discouraging destructive behaviors, the therapist models more appropriate behavior and demonstrates strength and concern for the patient (Appelbaum and Levy 2002). As the patient's injurious behaviors and level of emotional intensity diminish, the patient can identify with the reflective function and mentalizing ability of the therapist. This can help the patient make better sense of his or her own subjective states and mental processes, as well as those of others.

Appelbaum and Levy (2002) pointed out that the supportive therapist strives to establish an arousal level in the patient optimal for learning, fostering a sense of self, and appreciating the consequences of behavior. These factors help to address ego and adaptive dysfunction in patients with borderline personality disorder. With such patients, the therapist works to create a sense of safety so as to reduce maladaptive defenses, which are typically linked to fears of annihilation, abandonment, and humiliation. Creating a sense of safety can help the patient begin to develop a more integrated sense of self and other in the context of reduced anxiety. Nevertheless, this sense of safety must be created without fostering regression, which can escalate those behaviors that the therapist is trying to address and reduce. Maladaptive or immature defenses, such as regression, denial, or projection, are not supported. As in much of supportive psychotherapy, the therapist tries to maintain a balance of supportive and expressive techniques.

An advance in the treatment of borderline personality disorder was the development of dialectical behavior therapy (DBT), which initially focused on reducing parasuicidal behavior (Linehan 1993; Linehan et al. 1994). Although this practical, multicomponent approach to therapy with borderline patients has been presented as an evolution of cognitive-behavioral therapy, certain main components of the treatment are decidedly supportive, in that they directly address ego function and adaptive skills. The open and explicit collaboration between patient and therapist on here-and-now issues in DBT is consistent with the style of supportive therapy. In particular, the use of mindfulness exercises is a direct measure that addresses both ego functioning and adaptive skill in teaching patients to develop intrapsychic distance from overwhelming emotional distress. In addition, DBT makes liberal use of slogans and sayings that reframe patients' isolated experience into shared experiential wisdom and that serve as feedback for validating both subjective states and real responsibility (Palmer 2002). Interestingly, a year-long clinical trial comparing DBT, transference-focused psychotherapy, and supportive psychotherapy demonstrated that those receiving supportive psychotherapy had significant positive changes in depression, anxiety, global functioning, and social adjustment. Compared with the DBT group, the supportive psychotherapy group had significant reductions in anger, but supportive psychotherapy was less effective in reducing suicidality, which is not surprising given the specific focus of DBT on parasuicidal behavior (Clarkin et al. 2007).

Substance Use Disorders

Substance use disorders are among the most common mental disorders (Hasin and Grant 2015). In the past, most psychiatry residents did not treat patients presenting with substance use disorders unless the patients presented with co-occurring psychiatric disorders (see the section "Co-Occurring Mental Illness and Substance Use Disorders" later in this chapter). Generally, residents learned about withdrawal syndromes and detoxification while working on inpatient psychiatric units that admitted patients with psychiatric disorders or substance-induced mental disorders. In contrast, current residency training in psychiatry involves at least 1 month of full-time clinical work with patients who have substance use disorders; thus, residents must learn about basic psychotherapeutic and medication management of these patients.

Pharmacotherapy

There are relatively few pharmacotherapies that are effective for substance use disorders, and these pharmacotherapies work best in the context of psychosocial treatment. Therefore, psychotherapy is an important intervention for substance use disorders. Some medications approved for use in substance use disorders are maintenance medications for opioid use disorder, such as methadone and buprenorphine (Fudala et al. 2003; Kleber 2003); aversive medications for maintenance of abstinence for alcohol use disorder, such as disulfiram (Fuller et al. 1986); heavy drinking and craving reducers, such as naltrexone (O'Malley et al. 1992; Volpicelli et al. 1992); or anticonvulsants such as topiramate that both support abstinence and reduce episodes of craving and heavy drinking (Blodgett et al. 2014).

To conduct psychotherapy with substance-using patients, the therapist must understand the psychopharmacology of classes of drugs that are commonly used nonmedically, typical presentations of intoxication and withdrawal, and the natural course of drug effects. The therapist also needs to be familiar with common or street knowledge about the drugs, including slang names and prices (Rounsaville and Carroll 1998). A good working knowledge of these drugs and the lifestyle of the patient who uses them can help the therapist begin to build a therapeutic alliance with the patient.

Treatment Principles

In the past, individual expressive treatments were the standard intervention for substance use disorders. Over time, it became clear that use of uncovering psychotherapy as a sole mode of treatment for substance use disorders was generally not effective. Other treatment approaches, such as group therapies, pharmacotherapies (e.g., methadone maintenance), and therapeutic communities, became mainstays of addiction treatment. Rounsaville and Carroll (1998) underscored the rationale for supportive psychotherapy when they described the reasons that expressive treatments, when offered as the sole ambulatory treatment, are not well suited to the needs of patients with substance use disorders. In expressive treatments, symptom control and development of coping skills are often not the primary focus. Patients drop out frequently because of a lack of focus on the patient's presenting problem and because patients find the therapist's neutral, abstaining stance anxiety provoking. Today, it is understood that interpretations of addictive behaviors are not sufficient to stop the addictive process and that increasing the patient's anxiety early in the treatment of a substance use disorder is likely to trigger a relapse. Therefore, the therapist should embark on a more uncovering type of treatment only when the patient has established a concrete method for maintaining abstinence or is being treated within a protected environment (Brill 1977; Rosenthal and Westreich 1999).

Supportive psychotherapy with patients who have substance use disorder focuses on helping patients to develop effective coping strategies to control or reduce substance use and stay engaged in treatment. Other important components of treatment are developing and maintaining a strong therapeutic alliance and minimizing the risk of relapse by helping the patient to both reduce and learn to manage anxiety and dysphoria. Because supportive psychotherapy offers a broad and flexible foundation for interventions with patients, work with addicted patients typically includes use of newer, more evidence-based strategies, such as motivational interviewing, relapse prevention, and psychoeducation. General supportive principles are maintained during the course of addiction treatment, even as patient and therapist embark on particular cognitive and behavioral work, such as building cognitive skills. For a patient with a substance use disorder, individual supportive psychotherapy is often augmented and supported by the patient's engagement in a 12-step program, group therapy for substance use disorders, and other recovery-oriented therapeutic activities.

Motivational Interviewing

If an individual is not interested in reducing or stopping the use of substances when he or she meets the criteria for a substance use disorder, the individual may have a diagnosis but is not yet a patient. People who come into treatment for substance use disorders typically have spent months to years without severe consequences and have experienced drug use as fun or beneficial. People generally show up for substance use treatment only when the consequences of drug use have become threatening to their relationships, employment, health, freedom, or life. When these people then show up for treatment, most have beliefs about their drug use that were constructed when their use appeared to be free of severe negative consequences. A common belief is that drugs have played an essential role in the individual's ability to cope (Rounsaville and Carroll 1998). In this context, unless the patient sees the substance use as a problem and can conceptualize getting along without drug use, setting appropriate treatment goals is difficult.

Rollnick and Miller (1995) described motivational interviewing as a directive, patient-centered intervention that helps patients to explore and resolve their ambivalence about changing. The main principles of motivational interviewing include understanding the patient's view accurately, avoiding or deescalating resistance, and increasing the patient's self-efficacy and perception of the discrepancy between actual and ideal behavior (Miller and Rollnick 1991). Motivational interviewing is explicitly empathic and does not involve a coercive therapist position with respect to the patient's actions about reducing or stopping substance use; the patient might experience such a position as demeaning and damaging to self-esteem. A premise of motivational interviewing is that patients can decide to make changes on the basis of their own shifts in motivation. The techniques of motivational interviewing include listening reflectively and eliciting motivational statements from a patient, examining both sides of the patient's ambivalence, and reducing resistance by monitoring patient readiness and not pushing for change prematurely (Miller and Rollnick 1991). When the patient experiences that the negative consequences of substance use outweigh the positives ones, the so-called decisional balance is tipped in favor of engagement in treatment.

The respectful, collaborative, and empathic style of both motivational interviewing and supportive psychotherapy supports the development of a positive and healthy relationship that can reinforce reduction or cessation of substance use (Miller and Rose 2010). The supportive technique of clarifying the patient's role expectations and therapist's objectives and rationale early in treatment is advisable because discrepancy between role expectations and experiences in therapy may correlate negatively with alliance in patients with substance use disorders (Frankl et al. 2014).

PATIENT: OK, so I'll come in every week and you'll tell me what I should work on *(patient demonstrates expectation of a passive role in therapy)*.

THERAPIST: Not exactly. It sounds like you're expecting to have a more directed experience here, like in a classroom where the teacher lectures you and maybe gives you homework assignments *(uses metaphor to clarify meaning of prior statement)*.

PATIENT: What's wrong with that? Aren't you are the addiction expert? *(deflects and challenges)*

THERAPIST: Nothing is wrong with that *(doesn't argue)*.

PATIENT: I thought you'd figure out what's wrong with me and fix it *(restates the passive role expectation)*.

THERAPIST: Well, actually, we're both going to try to better understand your problems with substances, and then we'll collaborate on setting your goals and helping you meet them. There will be plenty of opportunity for me to give you information sometimes, but mostly you'll be learning through your community support services and online sites I recommend. I'll present my clinical objectives to you so we can discuss them. But this is important: if you're working actively with me and you feel responsible to pursue the goals that make sense to you, you're more likely to have a better outcome here *(informs about approach; supports agency)*.

Substantial evidence supports motivational interviewing as an effective intervention for substance use disorders—especially with regard to promoting entry into and engagement in more intensive treatments for substance use—even when the technique is used by clinicians who are not specialists in substance use treatment (Dunn et al. 2001). Therefore, motivational interviewing is a mainstay of supportive treatment of substance use disorders.

Adaptive Skills and Relapse Prevention

The main content of supportive treatment of substance use disorders is the work of achieving and maintaining abstinence from substances of abuse. Patients must learn new strategies that assist them in coping with craving states, negative emotions, general stress, and cues in the environment that serve as high-risk triggers for substance use. Long ago, the proponents of Alcoholics Anonymous identified exposure to the people, places, and things associated with alcohol use as a primer to relapse. A commonly heard maxim is that stopping the use of drugs is relatively easy, but remaining drug-free is hard. The specific adaptive skills that must be learned in addiction recovery are 1) identifying high-risk situations and cues, 2) anticipating exposure to these situations and cues, and 3) developing alternative strategies for coping when exposed to these situations.

Relapse prevention involves a formal set of cognitive-behavioral approaches to maintaining abstinence that are easily woven into supportive treatment. In relapse prevention, a systematic effort is made to identify the patient's specific relapse triggers and to devise and have the patient practice alternative behaviors and coping skills to deal with these triggers, such as refusal skills for when the patient is offered the target substance (Marlatt and Gordon 1985). However, identification of risky situations and development of coping skills to address these situations can also be done in a less structured fashion in supportive and supportive-expressive psychotherapy (Luborsky 1984). In any case, anticipatory guidance, encouragement, and reassurance are key supportive techniques that are used when identifying and rehearsing skills to cope with an expected situation. The therapist works to establish achievable intermediate goals, which help to reduce the risk of failure and of further damage to the patient's self-esteem.

When the patient reports that he or she has successfully negotiated some element of a high-risk situation, praise from the therapist related to the patient's goals is meaningful and reinforces the improvement in adaptive skills. The patient should already have experienced some increase in self-esteem through an experience of competence in achieving a life skill. If the patient tries but does not succeed, some praise is indicated because the patient tried to implement the adaptive skill. After some problem solving together, the therapist encourages the patient to try the skill again and reassures him or her about doing so. Thus, progress in executing new skills may be incremental, and the therapist offers measured but increasingly intense praise and positive feedback for each successive goal met.

Because a dysphoric mood is a frequently reported antecedent of relapse, the supportive treatment of substance use disorders also must focus on building adaptive skills for coping with negative or painful mood states (Marlatt and Gordon 1980). Substance-using individuals often have a difficult time differentiating mood states into specific affects, in part perhaps because they use the drugs to self-medicate dysphoria rather than developing psychological means to cope with the painful affects (Keller et al. 1995; Khantzian 1985). Therefore, therapists need to help patients with substance use disorder begin to reduce alexithymia in distinguishing one feeling from another. As Misch (2000) described, the ability to identify and label feelings makes it easier to reflect on these feelings and communicate about them to others. If the patient cannot notice and discriminate feelings, he or she cannot make clear connections between those feelings and the thoughts, behaviors, or events linked to drug use. For example, if patients cannot recognize when they are irritable and sad, they will not be able to connect either state to the automatic thoughts that they generate in response (e.g., "I'm feeling irritated, so I must get a bottle"). The ability to label feelings is essential for developing appropriate adaptive skills to manage painful affects. As patients begin to identify these feelings, they experience—in spite of increased awareness of negative affect—an increase in self-esteem that comes from mastery of the internal environment. The affects begin to be reframed as useful tools in identifying risky states that set up patients for relapse.

Psychoeducation

In the area of substance use disorders, education efforts focus on teaching patients about different classes of abused drugs, psychological and physical effects of drugs, dangers of chronic abuse, the fact that drugs may be used to self-medicate, and a disease model of addiction. Most cultures implicitly or explicitly operate out of a moral model of substance abuse and addiction, which attributes the irresponsible or criminal behavior of the addicted individual to his or her bad character. In contrast, the unitary disease concept of addiction, variously attributed to Alcoholics Anonymous (1976) or Jellinek (1952), stresses that addiction is a chronic, relapsing, and progressive illness. Furthermore, the advocates of the disease concept thought it was a mistake to think of alcoholism as a symptom of another disorder, such that if an underlying conflict were resolved in expressive treatment, the patient would stop drinking (Rosenthal and Westreich 1999). Jellinek's approach to alcoholism was not actually so reductionistic; he in fact described several typologies, which differed regarding onset, severity, pattern, and chronicity of use. Nonetheless, the psychotherapeutic utility of this heuristic approach is that it increases self-esteem by offering the patient a diagnosis rather than blame, helps the patient to cope better with shame (given that most patients presume that the moral model explains their own behavior), and offers another framework in which to foster a therapeutic alliance.

The following vignette illustrates the use of psychoeducation with a patient who uses substances nonmedically (see Video Vignette 6, available at www.appi.org/Winston).

Video Vignette 6: Substance Use Disorder

Kevin Waters is a 28-year-old single man who studied structural engineering in college but is currently unemployed, having been fired from his most recent of a string of jobs over the last few years, since he began using cocaine. He typically gets caught up in cocaine bingeing and fails to show up or notify his place of employment, with predictable results. He was living with his younger sister, her husband, and their 2-year-old daughter but was told to leave when he returned after a 3-day cocaine binge. He comes to the session full of regret and self-recrimination, a strong sense of the moral failure he has been given as feedback from both employers and family, and hopelessness.

In other cases, when a patient has less awareness of the negative consequences of his or her substance use, a therapist might rely more strongly on motivational interviewing techniques in the early phases (including nonjudgmental feedback to help the patient connect cause and effect) to assist the patient in deciding that his substance dependence is not worth what it costs in his life. In this session, the therapist instead uses psychoeducation to address Kevin's denial and uses a moral model to explain his addictive behavior. Because the moral model is intrinsically disempowering, which decreases self-esteem, the objective is that Kevin understand the disease concept and recognize that the loss of control is an inherent quality of substance dependence. Kevin may then feel more empowered to make decisions that incorporate that reality rather than channeling his energy into the self-blaming and unfruitful behavior that typically precedes or sustains a relapse.

> KEVIN: I can't stop the crack. I got thrown out of the house. I got no job, I got no money, I got no girl. I got nothing, except crack. I've blown up my life [*sighs, looks at therapist*]. Maybe they're right. Maybe I'm just no good [*looks down, shakes head, tears up*] **(attributes his drug-related losses and maladaptive behavior to being a bad person)**.
>
> THERAPIST: I know that the pain you're in right now makes you want to just blame yourself. And you've got a lot of reasons to feel bad right now. But can I ask you to consider your intentions for just a moment? It's important, but it will take a bit of reflection **(Empathically focuses patient away from self-blame to cognition)**.
>
> KEVIN: OK.
>
> THERAPIST: If you knew then what you know now—that your use results in the way your life is right now and the way you feel now—would you have done it anyway? **(clarification)**
>
> KEVIN: I don't think so. No, of course not. I wouldn't have done this if I had known…. No. **(takes rational position)**
>
> THERAPIST: So, what I'm saying to you is that your situation is predictable. This is what happens to people who become addicted to crack. Addiction is like a runaway train: Once you get on board, you don't necessarily go where you want the train to go. You go where the train takes you **(generalizes to others who have the same well-described problem; offers teaching metaphor)**.
>
> KEVIN: Yeah, but I'm the one who keeps doing it. I'm the one who started this up. I'm the one who doesn't stop. Like there's something's wrong with me! I'm stupid! **(retreats to moral model explanation; holds on to denial of loss of control)**
>
> THERAPIST: Well, I guess blaming yourself gives you some sense that you're still in control of this situation and that it's OK, when clearly it's not.
>
> KEVIN: I don't understand.
>
> THERAPIST: Well, let me put it this way: If you were stupid and couldn't learn, then that would explain the situation, but you're not stupid. You studied engineering successfully in college. Right? **(confronts distortion in self-description; builds alliance**

through demonstrating knowledge of patient's personal history)

KEVIN: Yeah, OK. So, I'm not stupid-stupid, but I've done such stupid stuff! [*scowls*] Maybe my sister is right; maybe I'm just weak and selfish *(acknowledges distortion but retreats to a different form of self-blame)*.

THERAPIST: So you just told me that if you knew then what you know now, you would not have made the same choices, and that now you're in a position where you can't stop. That's why we call it a disease. Loss of control comes with the territory; it's part of the disease. Drugs are powerful that way *(confronts denial, which is maladaptive for this patient, and offers a different explanation)*.

KEVIN: I understand what you're saying, but you might be saying this just to make me feel better—and that's fine—but I've got the rest of the world telling me I'm a waste of skin. I appreciate that, but...

THERAPIST: Let me show you something. These are the criteria for substance dependence in DSM [substance use disorder in DSM-5]. What you see here is that loss of control is one of the major symptoms. Right? [*opens to criteria for substance use disorder and points to the text while reading out loud*] "The substance is often taken in larger amounts or over a longer period than was intended. There is a persistent desire or unsuccessful efforts to cut down or control substance use" (American Psychiatric Association 2013a, p. 483) *(uses props, if necessary, to concretize the ideas and demonstrate expertise)*.

KEVIN: Huh. So I've tried so many times to just do only some, but I always spend everything I have *(recognizes own loss of control; becomes sad)*.

THERAPIST: So, maybe initially when you started, you made the mistake of thinking that you could get away with just using, but that was a long time ago. Things are a little different now. What you have now is called a disorder. Addiction and alcoholism are things that run in families. They are inherited. The risk is inherited, and drug problems are very similar *(supports patient's understanding with clarification, normalizing, rationalizing, and new knowledge)*.

KEVIN: My dad was an alcoholic. So was my uncle. I think that's what killed my uncle *(confirms understanding that his problems are more than about just willpower)*.

THERAPIST: So, that's my point. It's not your fault—but maybe now you understand that you and I must work together in order to help you fight this disease *(sides with the patient against the disease; supports the need for collaboration)*.

KEVIN: It just seems impossible. Do you think I really can get help with this? *(elicits reassurance)*

THERAPIST: I know it seems that way now, particularly when you recognize the loss of control, but this is a very common experience for people who are in the early stages or in the beginnings of recovery. But those who stay with treatments tend to have better outcomes than those who don't stay with treatments *(offers empathic reassurance based on expert knowledge, normalizing)*.

KEVIN: I hope you're right.

THERAPIST: I know right now it seems like there's a very long way to go. This is going to be difficult, but addiction is a treatable illness, like many other chronic illnesses. We don't have a cure for diabetes. We don't have a cure for hypertension. But people are able to recover from the more severe forms of the illness. Even with the illness being out of control, they can go on to have better lives *(expert opinion, normalizing, and offering reassurance)*.

Co-occurring Mental Illness and Substance Use Disorders

Prevalence and Treatment

About half of the population with severe mental disorders is affected by substance use disorders (Regier et al. 1990). Clinical samples of psychiatric patients often have higher than usual rates of alcohol use disorders and other substance use disorders (Fernandez-Pol et al. 1988; Fischer et al. 1975; Galanter et al. 1988; Richard et al. 1985). In the National Comorbidity Survey, Kessler et al. (1994) found that of the population who had psychosis or mania or who needed hospitalization for a mental disorder in a 12-month period, almost 90% met the criteria for three or more lifetime alcohol or drug use disorders or mental disorders.

Co-occurrence of substance use and other mental disorders has a negative effect on the trajectory of and recovery from both disorders (Rosenthal and Westreich 1999). Because patients with substance use disorders and schizophrenia are difficult to engage in treatment, supportive psychotherapy, with its focus on building and maintaining a therapeutic alliance, is a good treatment approach for this population (Carey et al. 1996; Lehman et al. 1993). Supportive treatment for those with both disorders integrates the techniques that are useful for each problem, as delineated in the sections "Severe Mental Illness" and "Substance Use Disorders" earlier in this chapter. Improving adaptive skills by increasing competence in basic conversational and recreational skills, using medication and symptom management, and using relapse prevention for negotiating situations likely to trigger relapse to substance abuse are all generally needed to treat co-occurring substance use disorders and other mental illnesses. Implementing these interventions has a beneficial effect on treatment retention and substance use in patients with psychotic illness and substance use disorders (Ho et al. 1999). Multiple studies have shown that psychosocial treatment that integrates psychiatric and addiction treatment components leads to better retention and better outcome among patients with severe mental illness and substance use disorders (Drake et al. 2001; Hellerstein et al. 1995).

Additional factors that work in concert with individual supportive treatments are support for patient involvement in 12-step programs (especially programs that are less likely to reduce self-esteem, such as "double trouble" or dual recovery groups) and family psychoeducation. In addition to praise, support for access to concrete services, socialization, recreation, and other opportunities can serve as positive reinforcement for attendance and may support the development of a therapeutic alliance and the engagement of patients in treatment (Rosenthal et al. 2000).

Psychoeducation

In the context of supportive treatment, patients with substance use disorders and mental illness should be given information about both classes of disorders. Like other supportive techniques, psychoeducation must be formulated in the context of the therapist's appraisal of the patient's capacity to make use of the information in a way that supports ego function or adaptive skills. For example, when a patient with a severe mental illness learns that he or she has another chronic illness such as substance dependence, this knowledge can become a factor in his or her demoralization (Rosenthal and Westreich 1999). The therapist teaches about both the substance dependence and the other mental illness: their symptoms, treatment, and natural history. Patients are encouraged to discuss their own symptoms and their own history of treatment responsiveness and to attempt to understand what role their substance abuse may have played in either relieving or exacerbating psychotic, mood, and anxiety symptoms.

Most patients with co-occurring substance use disorders and severe mental disorders who come into contact with treatment systems are not motivated to stop the use of substances. With these patients, motivational interviewing techniques can be useful within the context of supportive psychotherapy (Ziedonis and Fisher 1996; Ziedonis and Trudeau 1997). The process of recovery in patients with comorbid substance use disorders and other mental disorders is not linear, and exacerbation of both disorders is episodic. Patients may cycle repeatedly through different phases of treatment—engagement, active treatment, maintenance, relapse, and then reengagement. When patients come back into contact with treating clinicians after a relapse, they may be in an earlier motivational stage; they may even be in denial that a substance abuse problem exists (Prochaska and DiClemente 1984). Motivational techniques, which are traditionally used at the beginning of therapy to engage patients with substance use disorder in treatment, are thus used as a continuing component of supportive treatment for patients with co-occurring substance use disorders and severe mental illness. This approach is needed because patients cycle between motivational levels, with the various flare-ups of substance use disorders and other mental illness over time (Rosenthal and Westreich 1999). The time frame of recovery from substance use disorders is longer for patients with dual diagnoses than for patients without comorbid severe mental disorders. If a patient remains in treatment, however, reduction in severity of both disorders is a realistic prospect (Drake et al. 1993; Hellerstein et al. 1995).

Conclusion

Supportive psychotherapy provides a broad basic platform for psychotherapeutic intervention; therefore, treatment strategies and approaches such as motivational interviewing, psychoeducation, and relapse prevention, which are typically associated with specific clinical subpopulations, can be readily implemented in the context of treatment with supportive psychotherapy. In patients with personality disorders, supportive psychotherapy has beneficial impact and can serve as a natural platform for integrating other treatment strategies (e.g., using dialectical behavior therapy for patients with borderline personality disorder). In populations such as those with co-occurring substance use and other mental disorders, the alliance-building strategies of supportive psychotherapy plus motivational techniques can be applied over time to help maintain the patient's engagement in treatment through cycles of relapse and recovery.

Evaluating Competence and Outcome Research

9

The Accreditation Council for Graduate Medical Education (ACGME) defined six areas of competence for medical trainees: 1) patient care, 2) medical knowledge, 3) practice-based learning and improvement, 4) interpersonal and communication skills, 5) professionalism, and 6) systems-based practice (Accreditation Council for Graduate Medical Education 2014). Although outlining and describing areas of competence are within grasp at the present time, the tasks of defining, evaluating, and measuring competence of trainees are more complex. Development of measurement tools and their application to specific areas of competence is under way but still in an early stage.

The ACGME suggested a number of methods of measuring competence. These methods include various types of written, oral, and clinical examinations; a combined assessment approach of patient, family, supervisors, and others; record reviews; portfolios and case logs; simulations, models, and use of standardized patients; and evaluation of live or recorded performance (Accreditation Council for Graduate Medical Education 2015). The Residency Review Committee for Psychiatry chose five types of psychotherapy in which residents in psychiatry must be certified as competent by their training programs, but a few years later decreased this requirement to three types: supportive, psychodynamic (or, in our terminology, expressive), and cognitive-behavioral psychotherapies (Accreditation Council for Graduate Medical Education 2014). In this chapter, we outline our approach to evaluating competence of psychiatry trainees in one of these three psychotherapies—namely, supportive psychotherapy.

The definition of competence is a major issue that needs to be addressed. An acceptable definition of competent is "having requisite or adequate ability or qualities" (*Merriam-Webster's Collegiate Dictionary*, 11th Edition). Epstein and Hundert (2002) defined *professional competence* as "the habitual and judicious use of communication, knowledge, technical skills, clinical reasoning, emotions, values, and reflection in daily practice for the benefit of the individual and community being served" (p. 226). In assessments of psychotherapy trainees, supervisors should look for competence, not a high level of expertise (Manring et al. 2003).

When addressing a resident's competence, it is necessary to define what will be assessed and the method or methods of assessment. The evaluation process should be educational and promote resident learning. Professional competence can be conceptualized as a continuum of levels of ability or skill, from beginner to competent to expert. A trainee would be expected to be competent and thus be at the middle of this continuum.

Research Studies on the Teaching of Psychotherapy

There are a few relatively recent research studies on the teaching of psychotherapy. Truong et al. (2015) identified and evaluated studies on teaching psychotherapy to psychiatry residents and medical students. They found nine studies, but only one trial was judged to be methodologically rigorous. They called for additional well-designed studies to evaluate the teaching of psychotherapy to trainees.

Sudak and Goldberg (2012) reported their findings of a survey of U.S. general psychiatry training directors about the amount of didactic training and supervised clinical experience and the number of patients treated in the models of psychotherapy mandated by the Residency Review Committee for Psychiatry. They found expressive psychotherapy training to be the most robust, with the greatest variability, and training in cognitive-behavioral therapy was found to have advanced significantly. Supportive psychotherapy was the most widely practiced but received the least amount of didactic time and supervision.

Feinstein et al. (2015), at the University of Colorado, opted to teach psychiatric residents about the common factors in psychotherapy that positively affect psychotherapy outcomes. However, they did not study how learning about common factors enables residents to produce better psychotherapy outcome results. Gastelum et al. (2013) proposed an integrated approach for teaching psychodynamic psychotherapy to trainees in which uncovering and supportive techniques are taught side by side with specific guidelines for assessing when to use one set of interventions or the other. Unfortunately, they did not describe or propose a study to evaluate this approach.

As can be gleaned from these few studies, there are essentially no methodologically sound studies of psychotherapy teaching. Therefore, in the next few pages we will describe our approach to psychotherapy teaching and supervision, which is based on the American Association of Directors of Psychiatric Residency Training competencies for supportive psychotherapy. We believe that our approach is in keeping with the teaching of the core clinical principles of supportive psychotherapy, which is accepted at most psychiatry teaching programs.

Psychotherapy Supervision

Assessment of residents' competence in psychotherapy is an ongoing process in many residency programs. Evaluations of residents are performed by clinical supervisors during the process of psychotherapy supervision and are formally discussed with the residents one or more times a year.

Clinical supervision, as well as more formal seminars and classroom teaching, has long been a part of psychotherapy training. Seminars and classroom approaches generally consist of reading courses, in which psychotherapy theory and practice are taught, and clinical case seminars, which focus on evaluation, case formulation, diagnosis, and ongoing psychotherapy. Many training programs in psychiatry have established traditions of intensive individual supervision of residents, particularly in long-term expressive (exploratory) psychotherapy. The process of supervision may vary from one program to another but generally involves the following:

1. Presentation of the case by the resident
2. Discussion of the diagnosis, case formulation, goals, and treatment plan
3. Ongoing summary of sessions by the resident, using an informal recall-and-summary approach, process notes, video recordings, or a combination of these approaches
4. Discussion of the psychotherapy process, including resistance, dysfunctional thinking, defenses, affect, and therapist interventions, as well as

dynamics, genetics, psychological structure, cognitive-behavioral issues, and the therapeutic relationship (transference, countertransference, and the therapeutic alliance)

The supervisor has traditionally evaluated the resident's work by noting how well the resident performs the tasks listed above, as well as assessing other areas such as the ability to listen and relate to the patient in an empathic manner. The evaluation process by the supervisor is ongoing, but formal evaluations are generally performed once or twice a year or more. The formal evaluations are based on material discussed by the trainee through the use of process notes. Traditionally, the entire process has been somewhat informal and rarely standardized. In this chapter, we propose a standardized evaluation approach, one based on the use of video recordings during an ongoing course of psychotherapy.

Assessment

Focus

Assessment of competence in supportive psychotherapy should be evaluated within the broader context of general psychotherapy. The assessment should encompass skills of, attitudes toward, and knowledge about general psychotherapy and the more specific approach of supportive psychotherapy. General psychotherapy skills, as described by the American Association of Directors of Psychiatric Residency Training (AADPRT) Psychotherapy Task Force (2000), include establishing and maintaining boundaries and the therapeutic alliance, listening, addressing emotions, understanding, using supervision, dealing with resistances and defenses, and applying intervention techniques. Beitman and Yue (1999) described a similar set of skills, which they called *core psychotherapy skills*. They included other skills, such as identifying patterns and implementing strategies for change. The AADPRT Psychotherapy Task Force also developed psychotherapy competencies for the five psychotherapies originally mandated by the Residency Review Committee for Psychiatry, including supportive psychotherapy. Table 9–1 includes the complete list of AADPRT competencies for supportive psychotherapy (Pinsker et al. 2001).

The supportive psychotherapy competencies are divided into knowledge about, skills of, and attitudes toward supportive psychotherapy. The knowledge category encompasses knowledge about objectives, the patient-therapist relationship, and indications and contraindications for supportive psychotherapy. The skills section contains 15 items, including the ability to maintain a therapeutic alliance, the ability to use appropriate interventions, and the ability to establish treatment goals. The attitudes sec-

---

Table 9–1. American Association of Directors of Psychiatric Residency Training competencies for supportive psychotherapy

---

Knowledge

1. The resident will demonstrate knowledge that the principal objectives of supportive therapy are to maintain or improve the patient's self-esteem, minimize or prevent recurrence of symptoms, and maximize the patient's adaptive capacities.

2. The resident will demonstrate understanding that the practice of supportive therapy is commonly used in many therapeutic encounters.

3. The resident will demonstrate knowledge that the patient-therapist relationship is of paramount importance.

4. The resident will demonstrate knowledge of indications and contraindications for supportive therapy.

5. The resident will demonstrate understanding that continued education in supportive therapy is necessary for further skill development.

Skills

1. The resident will be able to establish and maintain a therapeutic alliance.

2. The resident will be able to establish treatment goals.

3. The resident will be able to interact in a direct and nonthreatening manner.

4. The resident will be able to be responsive to the patient and give feedback and advice when appropriate.

5. The resident will demonstrate the ability to understand the patient as a unique individual within his or her family and sociocultural community.

6. The resident will be able to determine which interventions are in the best interest of the patient and will exercise caution about basing interventions on his or her own beliefs and values.

7. The resident will be able to recognize and identify affects in the patient and himself or herself.

8. The resident will be able to confront in a collaborative manner behaviors that are dangerous or damaging to the patient.

9. The resident will be able to provide reassurance to reduce symptoms, improve morale and adaptation, and prevent relapse.

10. The resident will be able to support, promote, and recognize the patient's ability to achieve goals that will promote his or her well-being.

11. The resident will be able to provide strategies to manage problems with affect regulation, thought disorders, and impaired reality-testing.

12. The resident will be able to provide education and advice about the patient's psychiatric condition, treatment, and adaptation while being sensitive to specific community systems of care and sociocultural issues.

Table 9–1. American Association of Directors of Psychiatric
Residency Training competencies for supportive
psychotherapy *(continued)*

---

13. The resident will be able to demonstrate that in the care of patients with chronic disorders, attention should be directed to adaptive skills, relationships, morale, and potential sources of anxiety or worry.
14. The resident will be able to assist the patient in developing skills for self-assessment.
15. The resident will be able to seek appropriate consultation and/or referral for specialized treatment.

Attitudes

1. The resident will be empathic, respectful, curious, open, nonjudgmental, collaborative, and able to tolerate ambiguity and display confidence in the efficacy of supportive therapy.
2. The resident will be sensitive to sociocultural, socioeconomic, and educational issues that arise in the therapeutic relationship.
3. The resident will be open to audiotaping, videotaping, or direct observation of treatment sessions.

Source. Pinsker et al. 2001.

tion includes an empathic, respectful, nonjudgmental approach and sensitivity to sociocultural, socioeconomic, and educational issues.

Method

Assessment of a trainee's competence in supportive psychotherapy can be accomplished using a number of different methodologies, including administration of written and/or oral examinations that test the resident's knowledge base, use of simulated patients reading from standardized scripts, the request that the resident respond to a patient vignette using a supportive approach, and a supervisor's evaluation of a resident performing supportive psychotherapy. A formal written evaluation of the resident by the supervisor should be completed at least twice a year. This evaluation should be educative and be based on the supervisory work preceding the formal evaluation. The supervisor should provide the resident with verbal feedback on a regular basis.

We have found that supervisor evaluations of ongoing, video-recorded psychotherapy sessions are the best method of teaching and evaluating residents. Video-recorded sessions enable the supervisor or resident evaluator to observe the conduct of psychotherapy directly. The more traditional method of summarizing a session or working from process notes is less likely to convey what actually occurred in a psychotherapy session, even under the best of circumstances. The availability of video recordings opens the process of psychotherapy to an outside observer and makes evaluation of therapy more objective.

Evaluation of video-recorded supportive psychotherapy sessions should begin with the resident's assessment of the patient and should continue throughout a patient's psychotherapy. Each supervision session should begin with a brief summary by the resident, followed by a review of the video recording. Because an entire video recording is likely too lengthy for review in a supervisory hour, the supervisor and resident must decide which segments to review. The choice of video segments for viewing can be made on the basis of the resident's summary, which may point to areas of difficulty or significance.

Having trainees view recordings of psychotherapy sessions conducted by others essentially replaces a supervisory experience and can be used to assess the trainee's knowledge level, which cannot always be equated with skill. This procedure allows for discussion of techniques and of the broad range of possible therapeutic interventions.

A number of questions have been raised about the feasibility of using video recordings of psychotherapy for supervision. Difficulties cited include the cost and maintenance of the equipment and the ability of residents to operate the recording equipment. The cost of video equipment has decreased in recent years, enabling many training programs to offer video recording to residents. Video equipment has become easy to operate, and residents are able to make good recordings. Therefore, it seems feasible for residency programs to provide video equipment for residency training in psychotherapy. In the event that video equipment cannot be provided by the institution, it would not be unreasonable to require each trainee to provide his or her own camera. After all, training programs generally do not provide each resident with textbooks. The main purpose of recording is not to have a high-quality picture but rather an understandable audio that runs without attention from the therapist for the entire session.

Some residency programs may not be ready to begin with evaluations involving video. The evaluation form presented in the following subsection can be used to evaluate a trainee reporting on psychotherapy sessions from process notes. Another approach would be to present a video recording or written material from a supportive psychotherapy session and ask the resident questions about the treatment plan, case formulation, goals, technique, alliance, and so on. In addition, the resident could be asked to respond to the patient's complaints using a supportive psychotherapy approach.

Assessment Instrument

The AADPRT supportive psychotherapy competencies provided the basis for our development of a rating form to be used as a measure of a resident's competence in supportive psychotherapy. Our form (Figure 9–1) does not include all the items on the AADPRT list of competencies because it would not be practical or reasonable for training programs to use lengthy evaluation forms for three different psychotherapies. In addition, we modified or combined some items with other items from the supportive psychotherapy and general psychotherapy competencies.

The evaluation form covers three areas: knowledge (general psychotherapy competencies), attitudes, and skills. The rating is on a Likert scale of 0–5 (0=can't say, 1=unsatisfactory, 2=approaching competence, 3=competent, 4=competent plus, 5=expert). The advantages of this evaluation form are that it can be scored and that it also includes space for the supervisor's comments. The final score is calculated by dividing the number of questions scored into the total score. An average score of 3 or better suggests that the resident has demonstrated competence in supportive psychotherapy. In addition, the supervisor should write some overall comments about the resident, including the resident's strengths and overall performance, the resident's ability to work in and use supervision, and areas needing further work. The supervisor should discuss the evaluation with the resident in a way that is supportive and promotes the resident's education.

Conferences in which supportive psychotherapy supervisors discuss the supervisory and evaluation processes are important because they help standardize the evaluation of competence in supportive psychotherapy. One method of achieving reliability would be to have groups of supervisors rate supportive psychotherapy video recordings and then discuss their ratings. Discussions would be directed at reaching a consensus in the evaluation ratings. This approach has been used in psychotherapy research to measure therapist adherence to manual-based forms of psychotherapy (Waltz et al. 1993).

Supervisors in the Beth Israel Medical Center Psychotherapy Training Program rated 51 residents on their supportive psychotherapy work using the Resident Evaluation for Competence in Supportive Psychotherapy (Figure 9–1). The vast majority of residents were rated as competent or better. More important, the form served as a useful supportive psychotherapy evaluation guide for both residents and supervisors, and the supervisors found the form to be useful and easy to use.

Resident Evaluation for Competence in Supportive Psychotherapy

Resident _____   Supervisor _____

Date _____   Period _____

Instructions: Please evaluate the resident's performance on the following items by entering the appropriate number on the scoring line after each item.

Can't say	Unsatisfactory	Approaching competence	Competent	Competent plus	Expert
0	1	2	3	4	5

Knowledge and attitudes   Score

1. The resident demonstrates knowledge that the principal objectives of supportive psychotherapy are to maintain or improve the patient's self-esteem, ameliorate or prevent recurrence of symptoms, improve psychological or ego functioning, and enhance adaptive capacities.   _____

2. The resident understands that supportive therapy is dynamically based and is part of a continuum ranging from supportive to expressive psychotherapy.   _____

3. The resident demonstrates knowledge that the patient-therapist relationship is of paramount importance and is not addressed unless it is negative.   _____

4. The resident demonstrates knowledge of indications and contraindications for supportive psychotherapy.   _____

5. The resident understands that appropriate boundaries (e.g., time, outside agencies and relationships, confidentiality, professional attitude) must be established and maintained.   _____

Skills   Score

1. The resident is able to establish and maintain a positive therapeutic alliance and interact with the patient in an empathic, respectful, direct, responsive, and nonthreatening manner.   _____

2. The resident relates to the patient in a conversational manner (i.e., does not interrogate or engage in passive listening).   _____

3. The resident is able to establish realistic and appropriate treatment goals.   _____

4. The resident uses supportive therapy interventions (clarification, confrontation, interpretation, advice, reassurance, encouragement, praise, rationalization, reframing) in an appropriate and timely manner.   _____

5. The resident is able to respect and strengthen adaptive defenses, distinguish between adaptive and maladaptive defenses, and work to minimize anxiety in an appropriate and timely manner.   _____

6. The resident provides education about the patient's psychiatric condition and medication, and if necessary, about community systems of care and ancillary treatments.   _____

Figure 9–1. Beth Israel resident evaluation form for competence in supportive psychotherapy.

7. The resident focuses on the patient's present-day life while not ignoring the past and consistently works at improving self-esteem, promoting adaptation and ego functions, and ameliorating symptoms. ____

Total score: ____

Divided by number of items scored: ____ = ____

Supervisor's comments *(include comments on overall performance, strengths, areas needing further work, and the ability to work in and use supervision):*

_____
_____
_____
_____

Resident's signature _____
(This evaluation was discussed with me.)

Supervisor's signature_____

Evaluation based on *(check all that apply)*
Weekly supervision ____ Review of psychotherapy video ____
Review of psychotherapy notes ____

Figure 9–1. Beth Israel resident evaluation form for competence in supportive psychotherapy. *(continued)*

Outcome Research

In this section we report on a number of clinical trials of supportive psychotherapy in the treatment of various psychiatric disorders. We discuss some early uncontrolled studies and more recent controlled trials that address the efficacy of supportive psychotherapy.

Menninger Psychotherapy Research Project

The psychotherapy research project of the Menninger Foundation was an important early study comparing supportive and expressive psychotherapy with psychoanalysis. Wallerstein (1986, 1989) studied the treatment, clinical course, and posttreatment follow-up of 42 inpatients at the Menninger Foundation. Findings included the following: psychoanalysis produced more limited outcomes than predicted, whereas psychotherapy including supportive psychotherapy often achieved more than predicted; all the treatments became more supportive during the course of therapy;

and supportive interventions accounted for more of the change in outcome. This study took a naturalistic approach, without control subjects or random assignment of subjects, but it was noteworthy in calling attention to the possible efficacy of supportive psychotherapy.

Schizophrenia Studies

In a National Institute of Mental Health study, patients with schizophrenia were treated for 2 years with either exploratory, insight-oriented psychotherapy three times a week or the control therapy (called reality-adaptive, supportive psychotherapy) once a week. Results provided clear evidence of a better outcome for patients treated with the supportive psychotherapy (Gunderson et al. 1984; Stanton et al. 1984). All patients were maintained on their usual medications throughout the study.

In another study, patients with schizophrenia were randomly assigned to supportive psychotherapy or family treatment (Rea et al. 1991). Patients were treated for 9 months and followed for 2 years. Supportive psychotherapy consisted of medication case management, crisis intervention, and education about schizophrenia, whereas family treatment involved problem-solving therapy and communication skills training. Patients in supportive treatment had significant improvement in coping style compared with patients in family therapy. However, the two groups were not at comparable levels of coping skills at initiation of treatment, and this fact was not considered in the statistical analysis.

Hogarty et al. (1997) stated that supportive psychotherapy fares less well compared with other psychosocial approaches, such as family psychoeducation, skills training, or role therapy. Defining supportive psychotherapy as not including psychoeducation, skills training, or role therapy approaches is problematic, however, because most therapists practicing supportive psychotherapy commonly employ these approaches. Other psychotherapy approaches with patients who have schizophrenia include social skills training, which may be enhanced with amplified skills training in the community (Glynn et al. 2002; Liberman et al. 1998).

A study in Copenhagen (Rosenbaum et al. 2012) compared supportive psychodynamic psychotherapy with treatment as usual, consisting of psychoeducation: meetings with psychologists and social workers; group meetings; and medical advice in patients with first-episode psychosis. They found that the supportive psychotherapy group improved significantly more than the treatment as usual group in social function and general psychopathology.

In another study of first-episode psychosis using supportive psychodynamic psychotherapy, Harder et al. (2014) found significant improvement on social functioning, overall symptoms, and positive psychotic symptoms. The improvement found was not sustained at 5-year follow-up. This finding is not surprising because most patients with psychotic disorders require long-term follow-up to prevent relapse.

In a randomized controlled trial for young people at ultra high risk of psychosis treated with cognitive therapy plus risperidone, cognitive therapy plus placebo, or supportive therapy plus placebo, McGorry et al. (2013) found that all groups improved substantially, particularly in terms of negative symptoms and overall functioning.

Depressive Disorder Studies

In the National Institute of Mental Health Treatment of Depression Collaborative Research Program, two psychotherapies (cognitive-behavioral therapy and interpersonal therapy) were compared with an antidepressant (imipramine)–clinical management condition and a control condition consisting of drug placebo and clinical management (Elkin 1994; Elkin et al. 1989; Imber et al. 1990). The clinical management was a low-level supportive psychotherapy approach. The two psychotherapies were found to be efficacious but not significantly different from the placebo–clinical management condition on measures of depressive symptoms and overall functioning.

Thompson and Gallagher (1985) studied 30 outpatients ranging in age from 60 to 81 years. Patients were randomly assigned to a 16-week treatment with cognitive therapy, behavior treatment, or supportive psychotherapy. Improvement was similar across the three treatment conditions at termination, but at 1-year follow-up, more of the patients in supportive psychotherapy received a diagnosis of depression. Unfortunately, the small number of patients in each treatment group and the type of supportive psychotherapy used make these findings of limited value.

In a randomized clinical trial involving 100 adolescents with depression, Renaud et al. (1998) compared cognitive, family, and supportive psychotherapies and found that rapid responders to therapy had better outcomes at 1-year follow-up and better scores on some measures at 2-year follow-up. The investigators concluded that their findings suggest that patients with milder forms of depression may benefit from initial supportive psychotherapy or short trials of more specialized types of psychotherapy.

Maina et al. (2005) completed a randomized controlled trial comparing brief dynamic therapy with supportive psychotherapy in treating patients with minor depressive disorders. Both therapies showed significant improvement in comparison with nontreated control subjects, but brief dynamic therapy was more effective at follow-up evaluation.

In a meta-analysis involving patients with major depression, de Maat et al. (2008) compared short-term psychodynamic supportive psychotherapy with antidepressant treatment and also with combined psychotherapy and medication. The results of the meta-analysis indicated that combined therapy is more efficacious than pharmacotherapy alone and that psychotherapy alone and pharmacotherapy alone seem equally efficacious.

Kocsis et al. (2009) compared a cognitive-behavioral analysis system of psychotherapy with brief supportive psychotherapy in their ability to augment antidepressant nonresponse in patients with chronic depression. Although 37.5% of subjects experienced partial response or remission, neither form of adjunctive psychotherapy improved outcome compared with a flexible, individualized pharmacotherapy regimen alone.

In a study comparing supportive psychotherapy and cognitive-behavioral therapy for the treatment of depression following traumatic brain injury, Ashman et al. (2014) found that both forms of psychotherapy were efficacious in improving diagnoses of depression and anxiety and reducing depressive symptoms.

Schramm et al. (2017) found that a specific form of cognitive-behavioral therapy for chronic depression had somewhat better outcome results than a nonspecific supportive psychotherapy. However, both forms of psychotherapy produced good results, and the supportive psychotherapy was not specific for depression.

Anxiety Disorder Studies

Systematic hierarchical desensitization was compared with supportive psychotherapy in a 26-week treatment trial involving patients with various types of phobias (Klein et al. 1983). Both treatments performed well, and no difference was found between the two approaches. The authors speculated that for individuals with phobia, psychotherapy serves as an instigator of corrective activity outside the formal session by maintaining exposure in vivo. In another study, patients with phobias and panic attacks received either imipramine plus behavior therapy or imipramine plus supportive psychotherapy (Zitrin et al. 1978). The majority of patients showed moderate to marked improvement, and there was no difference between behavior therapy and supportive psychotherapy in terms of improvement rates.

In a study of social anxiety disorder (phobia), Alström et al. (1984) found that supportive psychotherapy and prolonged exposure therapy were equally effective. Herbert et al. (2009) compared individual cognitive-behavioral therapy, group cognitive-behavioral therapy, and an educational-supportive psychotherapy that did not contain specific cognitive-behavioral therapy elements in treating patients with social anxiety disorder. They found that all three treatments produced significant reductions in symptoms and functional impairment, as well as improved social skills, with no differences between treatments.

In another study of social anxiety disorder, Lipsitz et al. (2008) found that supportive psychotherapy and interpersonal therapy produced significant improvement from pretreatment to posttreatment, with neither therapy being superior to the other. However, Shear et al. (2001) reported that emotion-focused psychotherapy, a form of supportive psychotherapy, has low efficacy for the treatment of panic disorder. They compared emotion-focused psychotherapy with cognitive-behavioral treatment, imipramine, or pill placebo in a study involving 112 subjects.

For studies on posttraumatic stress disorder, see the section on treatment approaches in Chapter 7, "Crisis Intervention."

Personality Disorder Studies

In a study comparing supportive with interpretive psychotherapy, Piper et al. (1998) found no outcome differences between the two treatments. Patients presented with anxiety or depressive disorders, and 60.4% of subjects had comorbid personality disorder. Hellerstein et al. (1998) compared brief supportive psychotherapy with short-term dynamic psychotherapy in treating patients with primarily Cluster C and not-otherwise-specified personality disorders, as well as comorbid disorders such as depression or anxiety. The authors reported similar efficacy on measures of symptomatology, presenting complaints, and interpersonal functioning. These changes were found not only at termination but also at 6-month follow-up. In a substudy of the study by Hellerstein et al. (1998), the authors used the Inventory of Interpersonal Problems mapped to an interpersonal circumplex model and graphically demonstrated lasting positive change in interpersonal functioning in the subjects treated with supportive psychotherapy (Rosenthal et al. 1999; Winston et al. 2001).

Clarkin et al. (2007) compared transference-focused psychotherapy, dialectical behavior therapy, and supportive psychotherapy in patients with borderline personality disorder and found significant positive change in multiple domains after one year of treatment. They suggested that these structured treatments for borderline personality disorder are generally equivalent with respect to broad positive change in these patients. In another study of borderline personality patients, Jørgensen et al. (2013) compared mentalization-based psychotherapy with supportive psychotherapy and found significant positive changes in both treatment groups on general functioning, depression, and social functioning.

Eating Disorder Studies

An evaluation of the efficacy of family-based treatment compared with supportive psychotherapy was undertaken by le Grange et al. (2007) for adolescent bulimia nervosa. Family-based treatment was found to have a clinical and statistical advantage over supportive psychotherapy.

Carter et al. (2011) examined the long-term efficacy of cognitive-behavioral therapy, interpersonal therapy, and specialist supportive clinical management in women with anorexia nervosa, with a mean follow-up of 6.7 years. They found no significant differences on outcome measures among the three psychotherapies at long-term follow-up, although supportive psychotherapy was associated with a more rapid response than interpersonal therapy.

Medical Disorder Studies

Mumford et al. (1982) reviewed controlled studies of supportive psychotherapy—including education about illness and treatments, cognitive-behavioral techniques, and venting and reassurance in a supportive relationship—in patients recovering from myocardial infarctions and surgery. The authors found that compared with patients receiving only typical medical care, patients receiving psychological intervention had better experiences with pain and increased patient compliance and speed of recovery, as well as fewer complications and fewer days in the hospital.

Conclusion

In this chapter, we have provided an overview of current efforts to evaluate the competence of residents engaged in various clinical tasks, and in particular supportive psychotherapy, as well as a summary of outcome research in supportive psychotherapy. We have presented a preliminary approach to evaluating psychiatry residents in supportive psychotherapy using an adaptation of the AADPRT list of supportive psychotherapy competencies. However, the process of evaluating competence is in an early phase of development and will require a great deal of reflection, planning, and study to achieve reliable and valid measurement systems. The brief review of the efficacy of supportive psychotherapy indicates that supportive treatment appears to be useful across a broad spectrum of psychiatric and medical disorders. However, more research is needed to clarify the indications for supportive psychotherapy and how this treatment should be integrated with other psychotherapy approaches and treatment with medication.

Questions for Self-Study

10

Items 1–7

Match each of the following items with the form of psychotherapy with which it is most closely aligned. Each item may be used once, more than once, or not at all.

A. Supportive psychotherapy
B. Expressive psychotherapy
C. Both supportive and expressive psychotherapy
D. Neither supportive nor expressive psychotherapy

___ 1. Aims to help a patient to cope with symptoms
___ 2. Aims to change a patient's fundamental personality
___ 3. Therapist plays an active and direct role
___ 4. Focuses on stability and adaptation
___ 5. The therapeutic relationship is important to the treatment process
___ 6. Focuses on resolution of unconscious conflict
___ 7. Its techniques are derived from a formal theory of mind

Items 8–10

Place each kind of therapeutic approach at the appropriate spot on the supportive-expressive continuum.

Supportive	A	Supportive	B	Expressive-	C
relationship		psychotherapy		supportive	
				psychotherapy	

___ 8. Psychoanalysis
___ 9. Counseling
___ 10. Supportive-expressive psychotherapy

Items 11–13

Identify the correct answer for each question.

___ 11. Which factor or combination of factors has been identified as common to most forms of effective psychotherapy?

    A. Atmosphere of warmth, hope, caring, and authenticity
    B. Clear theoretical framework
    C. Explicit and intense communication
    D. Frequent confrontation and limit setting
    E. Primary focus on behavior change

___ 12. Which of the following questions by a therapist is phrased in a manner that is least supportive of the self-esteem of the patient?

    A. What concerns do you have about your medication?
    B. What happened when you stopped taking your medication?
    C. When did you stop taking your medication?
    D. When have you found it helpful to take your medication?
    E. Why did you stop your medication?

___ 13. Which of the following are techniques associated with supportive psychotherapy?

    A. Advice, anticipatory guidance, naming the problem
    B. Avoidance of discussions of practical issues
    C. Cultivation of friendship between therapist and patient
    D. Frequent interpretation of transference issues
    E. Repeated self-disclosure by the therapist unrelated to patient needs

Items 14–16

Match each of the following descriptions with the concept with which it is most closely aligned. Each item may be used once, more than once, or not at all.

A. Advice
B. Confrontation
C. Education
D. Reassurance
E. Reframing

___ 14. The therapist saying, "You really should do regular exercise."
___ 15. The therapist saying, "Starting out slow with exercise is OK."
___ 16. The therapist saying, "Exercise is important to overall health and well-being."

Items 17–21

Match each of the following items with the form of psychotherapy with which it is most closely aligned. Each item may be used once, more than once, or not at all.

A. Supportive psychotherapy
B. Expressive psychotherapy
C. Both supportive and expressive psychotherapy
D. Neither supportive nor expressive psychotherapy

___ 17. Involves active two-way communication between therapist and patient
___ 18. Demonstrates respect for the patient as a person of worth and dignity
___ 19. Involves cultivation of friendship between therapist and patient
___ 20. Entails significant time and attention to the termination process
___ 21. May include adjuvant medication treatment

Items 22–25

Match each of the following descriptions with the concept with which it is most closely aligned. Each item may be used once, more than once, or not at all.

A. Advice
B. Confrontation

C. Education
D. Reassurance
E. Praise

___ 22. The therapist saying, "Don't quit your tennis team. Let's keep talking about it more before you decide."
___ 23. The therapist saying, "Based on what we've discussed, my impression is that your tennis partner will still want to remain friends if you make the decision to quit your tennis team."
___ 24. The therapist saying, "It seems like you can't handle the time demands of being on the tennis team."
___ 25. The therapist saying, "Transitioning from being on the tennis team—spending less time on the courts and giving more time to your studies and your relationship with your girlfriend—seems like a really positive step forward in your life."

Items 26–35

Identify the correct answer for each question.

___ 26. A 47-year-old woman seeks treatment 3 weeks after the sudden death of her husband of 22 years. She is often tearful, has difficulty sleeping, and feels worried about her future and the impact of their father's death on her teenage children. Which of the following is the most appropriate care?

A. Antidepressant medication
B. Benzodiazepine medication
C. Cognitive-behavioral therapy focused on negative cognitions
D. Long-term psychoanalytically oriented psychotherapy
E. Supportive therapy focused on grief and day-to-day coping

___ 27. Which of the following is necessary for supportive psychotherapy to be effective?

A. Abstinence from all substances
B. Completion of a comprehensive medical evaluation
C. Compliance with medication treatment
D. Willingness to attend psychotherapy sessions
E. Withdrawal from all other forms of psychotherapy (e.g., couples therapy)

___ 28. Which of the following patients is most likely to benefit from supportive psychotherapy?

A. A patient who has been found to be malingering
B. A patient who has been recently diagnosed with cancer
C. A patient who is actively suicidal
D. A patient with factitious disorder
E. A patient with signs of acute alcohol withdrawal

___ 29. Establishing firm ground rules for behaviors and expectations in therapy is especially important in supportive therapy involving patients living with which of the following personality disorders?

A. Borderline
B. Dependent
C. Histrionic
D. Narcissistic
E. Schizoid

___ 30. Which of the following is the most accurate statement regarding sexual involvement between a therapist and a patient in the context of supportive psychotherapy, according to the American Psychiatric Association and the American Psychological Association?

A. Always permitted
B. Never permitted
C. Not permitted while the patient is actively engaged in therapy
D. Permitted after the patient terminates the therapy
E. Permitted after the therapist terminates the therapy

___ 31. Examples of supportive psychotherapy techniques include which of the following?

A. Advice
B. Disclosure
C. Homework
D. Reassurance
E. All of the above

___ 32. Which of the following is the most accurate statement regarding self-disclosure by the therapist in the context of supportive psychotherapy?

A. Always permitted
B. Never permitted
C. Permitted when it serves to strengthen the therapeutic relationship or advance therapeutic goals
D. Permitted when the patient appears to enjoy the therapist's personal story
E. Permitted when the patient consents to this part of the therapy

___ 33. Examples of social skills that can be developed in the context of supportive psychotherapy include

A. Interviewing for a job
B. Making conversation and eye contact
C. Recognizing social cues
D. Rehearsing strategies for handling difficult situations
E. All of the above

___ 34. Which of the following may interfere with the effectiveness or slow down the process of supportive psychotherapy?

A. Addiction issues experienced by the patient
B. Aggressive feelings toward the therapist
C. Negative transferential feelings experienced by the patient
D. Psychotic symptoms of the patient
E. All of the above

___ 35. Supportive psychotherapy is likely to be ineffective in the context of which of the following conditions?

A. Adjustment disorders
B. Chronic medical conditions
C. Delirium
D. Early dementia
E. Substance use disorders

Items 36–42

Match each of the following descriptions with the concept with which it is most closely aligned. Each item may be used once, more than once, or not at all.

A. Supportive psychotherapy is valuable/indicated
B. Supportive psychotherapy may be valuable/indicated

C. Supportive psychotherapy is not valuable/indicated

D. Supportive psychotherapy is contraindicated

___ 36. Bereavement

___ 37. Factitious disorder

___ 38. Psychosis

___ 39. Depression

___ 40. "Baby blues"

___ 41. Locked-in syndrome

___ 42. Severe intellectual disability

Items 43–45

Identify the correct answer for each question.

___ 43. A 64-year-old man with long-standing bipolar disorder is encouraged by his family to speak with a therapist about the challenges he is facing as he moves to a nursing home/residential treatment setting after a recent hip replacement surgery. He has lived independently for many years but accepts that the new living arrangement will be helpful to him. Which of the following is the most accurate statement about the goals of supportive psychotherapy treatment?

A. The goals should align with the issues that are most important to the facility staff

B. The goals should align with the issues that are most important to the family

C. The goals should align with the issues that are most important to the patient

D. The goals should align with the issues that are most important to the patient's psychiatrist

E. The goals should align with the issues that are most important to the patient's surgeon

___ 44. A 28-year-old woman recently learned that she had been adopted at birth and sought psychotherapy to deal with her feelings of anger toward her biological parents and estrangement from her adoptive parents. Which of the following is the most accurate statement about the initial goals of the supportive psychotherapy treatment?

A. Treatment should be fully directed toward eliminating the patient's feelings of anger and estrangement

    B. Treatment should be fully directed toward issues other than the patient's feelings of anger and estrangement

    C. Treatment should fully focus on helping the patient cope with feelings of anger and estrangement

    D. Treatment should fully guarantee a reduction in feelings of anger and estrangement

    E. Treatment should fully replace feelings of anger and estrangement with feelings of joy and emotional connection

___ 45. An 18-year-old high school graduate feels unsettled by the prospect of attending college across the country in just a few months. Which of the following is the most accurate statement about psychotherapy in this context?

    A. Engaging in supportive psychotherapy for a few months is not likely to be beneficial

    B. Engaging in supportive psychotherapy in one state and then moving to another state is not likely to be beneficial

    C. Engaging in supportive psychotherapy focused on issues of separation and adaptation to the new college environment may be helpful

    D. Engaging in expressive psychotherapy with the goal of personality change is recommended in this situation

    E. Engaging in expressive psychotherapy with the goal of delaying the transition to college out of state is recommended in this situation

Items 46–50

Match each of the following descriptions with the concept with which it is most closely aligned. Each item may be used once, more than once, or not at all.

A. Supportive psychotherapy is valuable and is indicated as a first-line treatment

B. Supportive psychotherapy may be valuable and is indicated as a first-line or adjuvant treatment

C. Supportive psychotherapy is not valuable and is not indicated as a first-line treatment

D. Supportive psychotherapy is not valuable and is not indicated as a first-line or adjuvant treatment

E. Supportive psychotherapy is contraindicated as a first-line or adjuvant treatment

___ 46. An 18-year-old with new-onset psychosis who is acutely suicidal
___ 47. A 45-year-old with chronic schizoaffective disorder who is seeking employment
___ 48. A 65-year-old experiencing grief and significant depressive symptoms after the loss of a lifelong partner
___ 49. A 25-year old with opioid dependence who requests substance abuse detoxification
___ 50. A 35-year-old with symptoms of distress associated with gender dysphoria who has been bullied at work

Items 51–55

Identify the correct answer for each question.

___ 51. Supportive psychotherapy is conducted in which of the following communication styles?

A. Asymmetrical
B. Conversational
C. Formal
D. Oppositional
E. Technical

___ 52. Which of the following time frames is the focus of supportive psychotherapy with a middle-age adult?

A. Adolescence
B. Childhood
C. Future
D. Past 5 years
E. Present

___ 53. For patients engaged in supportive psychotherapy, ongoing goals of treatment should include which of the following?

A. Amelioration of symptoms
B. Enhancement of self-esteem
C. Improvement of adaptation to life circumstances
D. Improvement of overall functioning
E. All of the above

___ 54. Positive prognostic features associated with decreased potential for suicide include which of the following?

    A. Aggressivity
    B. Family support
    C. Hopelessness
    D. Pessimism
    E. Recent psychiatric hospitalization

___ 55. Supportive psychotherapy for acute bereavement may include which of the following?

    A. Concrete assistance with routine activities
    B. Diagnosis of underlying mental disorder affecting grief
    C. Emotional support
    D. Opportunity to express feelings of anger and loss
    E. All of the above

Items 56–59

Match each of the following descriptions with the concept with which it is most closely aligned. Each item may be used once, more than once, or not at all.

A. Anticipatory guidance
B. Confrontation
C. Expressions of empathy
D. Praise
E. Silence

___ 56. Therapeutic relationship-building technique
___ 57. Esteem-building technique
___ 58. Skill-building technique
___ 59. Behavioral pattern recognition-building technique

Items 60–64

Match each of the following descriptions with the type of psychosocial intervention or therapy with which it is most closely aligned. Each item may be used once, more than once, or not at all.

A. Crisis intervention
B. Supportive psychotherapy

C. Both crisis intervention and supportive psychotherapy
D. Neither crisis intervention nor supportive psychotherapy

___ 60. Typically provided as soon as possible
___ 61. Focuses only on "here and now" issues
___ 62. Uses silence as a primary technique
___ 63. Typically involves one-to-one therapy
___ 64. Focuses only on unconscious processes

Items 65–68

Match each of the following descriptions with the psychotherapeutic approach with which it is most closely aligned. Each item may be used once, more than once, or not at all.

A. Cognitive-behavioral approach
B. Dynamic approach
C. Genetic approach
D. Structural approach

___ 65. Focuses on fixed aspects of an individual's personality
___ 66. Focuses on early development experiences that influence the patient's current situation
___ 67. Focuses on current conflicts and their connection to primary or core psychological conflicts
___ 68. Focuses on automatic thoughts and how they can be changed to improve current life adaptation and behavior

Items 69–70

Identify the correct answer for each question.

___ 69. In supportive psychotherapy, treatment goals should *not*

A. Be defined mutually by the therapist and patient
B. Be documented in the patient's health record
C. Ever require adjuvant medication
D. Evolve during the course of therapy
E. Remain fixed and unchangeable over time

___ 70. Occasional lateness by a patient in supportive psychotherapy is handled by the therapist using

    A. A collaborative, problem-solving approach
    B. A confrontational approach
    C. An approach that focuses on addressing financial implications
    D. An approach that focuses on therapy termination
    E. An approach that focuses on unconscious conflicts

Items 71–75

Match each of the following descriptions with the concept with which it is most closely aligned. Each item may be used once, more than once, or not at all.

    A. Likely to benefit: appropriate candidate for supportive psychotherapy
    B. Uncertain: may or may not be appropriate candidate for supportive psychotherapy
    C. Not likely to benefit: not appropriate candidate for supportive psychotherapy

___ 71. Individuals with impaired reality testing
___ 72. Individuals with mild intellectual disability
___ 73. Individuals with psychotic symptoms
___ 74. Individuals with alexithymia
___ 75. Individuals with advanced dementia

Answers

1 C; 2 B; 3 A; 4 A; 5 C; 6 B; 7 C; 8 C; 9 A; 10 B; 11 A; 12 E; 13 A; 14 A; 15 D; 16 C; 17 A; 18 C; 19 D; 20 C; 21 C; 22 A; 23 D; 24 B; 25 E; 26 E; 27 D; 28 B; 29 A; 30 B; 31 E; 32 C; 33 E; 34 E; 35 C; 36 B; 37 C; 38 B; 39 B; 40 A; 41 C; 42 C; 43 C; 44 C; 45 C; 46 E; 47 B; 48 A; 49 B; 50 A; 51 B; 52 E; 53 E; 54 B; 55 E; 56 C; 57 D; 58 A; 59 B; 60 A; 61 A; 62 D; 63 C; 64 D; 65 D; 66 C; 67 B; 68 A; 69 E; 70 A; 71 B; 72 B; 73 B; 74 B; 75 C

References

Accreditation Council for Graduate Medical Education: The Psychiatry Milestone Project: Assessment Tools. Chicago, IL, Accreditation Council for Graduate Medical Education, 2014. Available at: August 29, 2019. Accessed August 29, 2019.

Accreditation Council for Graduate Medical Education: The Psychiatry Milestone Project. Chicago, IL, Accreditation Council for Graduate Medical Education, July 2015. Available at: www.acgme.org/Portals/0/PDFs/Milestones/PsychiatryMilestones.pdf?ver=2015-11-06-120520-753. Accessed August 29, 2019.

Adshead G: Murmurs of discontent: treatment and treatability of personality disorder. Adv Psychiatr Treat 7:407–417, 2001

Aguilera DC, Messick J, Farrel LM: Crisis Intervention. St. Louis, MO, Mosby, 1970

Alcoholics Anonymous: The Story of How Many Thousands of Men and Women Have Recovered From Alcoholism, 3rd Edition. New York, Alcoholics Anonymous World Service, 1976, p 12

Alexander F, French TM: Psychoanalytic Psychotherapy. New York, Ronald Press, 1946

Alström JE, Nordlund CL, Persson G, et al: Effects of four treatment methods on agoraphobic women not suitable for insight-oriented psychotherapy. Acta Psychiatr Scand 70(1):1–17, 1984 6147066

Alter CL: Palliative and supportive care of patients with pancreatic cancer. Semin Oncol 23(2):229–240, 1996 8623059

AMA Council on Ethical and Judicial Affairs: AMA Code of Medical Ethics' opinions on observing professional boundaries and meeting professional responsibilities. AMA J Ethics 17(5):432–434, 2015

American Association of Directors of Psychiatric Residency Training Psychotherapy Task Force: Psychotherapy Competencies. Farmington, CT, American Association of Directors of Psychiatric Residency Training, 2000

American Psychiatric Association: Diagnostic and Statistical Manual of Mental Disorders, 5th Edition. Washington DC, American Psychiatric Association, 2013a

American Psychiatric Association: The Principles of Medical Ethics With Annotations Especially Applicable to Psychiatry. Washington, DC, American Psychiatric Association, 2013b. Available at: www.psychiatry.org/File%20Library/Psychiatrists/Practice/Ethics/principles-medical-ethics.pdf. Accessed August 30, 2019.

American Psychological Association: Ethical Principles of Psychologists and Code of Conduct. Washington, DC, American Psychological Association, 2017. Available at: www.apa.org/ethics/code/index. Accessed August 30, 2019.

Appelbaum AH, Levy KN: Supportive psychotherapy for borderline patients: a psychoanalytic research perspective. Am J Psychoanal 62(2):201–202, 2002 12085529

Arnow BA, Steidtmann D, Blasey C, et al: The relationship between the therapeutic alliance and treatment outcome in two distinct psychotherapies for chronic depression. J Consult Clin Psychol 81(4):627–638, 2013 23339536

Artiss KL: Human behavior under stress: from combat to social psychiatry. Mil Med 128:1011–1015, 1963 14055063

Ashman T, Cantor JB, Tsaousides T, et al: Comparison of cognitive behavioral therapy and supportive psychotherapy for the treatment of depression following traumatic brain injury: a randomized controlled trial. J Head Trauma Rehabil 29(6):467–478, 2014 25370439

Balsam RM, Balsam A: Becoming a Psychotherapist: A Clinical Primer, 2nd Edition. Chicago, IL, University of Chicago Press, 1984

Bateman AW, Fonagy P: Effectiveness of psychotherapeutic treatment of personality disorder. Br J Psychiatry 177:138–143, 2000 11026953

Beck AT, Sokol L, Clark DA, et al: A crossover study of focused cognitive therapy for panic disorder. Am J Psychiatry 149(6):778–783, 1992 1590494

Beitman B, Yue D: Learning Psychotherapy: A Time-Efficient, Research-Based, and Outcome-Measured Training Program. New York, WW Norton, 1999

Bellack AS, Mueser KT: Psychosocial treatment for schizophrenia. Schizophr Bull 19(2):317–336, 1993 8322036

Bellak L: The schizophrenic syndrome: a further elaboration of the unified theory of schizophrenia, in Schizophrenia: A Review of the Syndrome. New York, Logos, 1958, pp 3–63

Beres D: Ego deviation and the concept of schizophrenia, in The Psychoanalytic Study of the Child, Vol 11. New York, International Universities Press, 1956, pp 164–235

Beutler LE, Moleiro C, Talebi H: Resistance in psychotherapy: what conclusions are supported by research. J Clin Psychol 58(2):207–217, 2002a 11793333

Beutler LE, Moleiro CM, Talebi H: Resistance, in Psychotherapy Relationships That Work: Therapist Contributions and Responsiveness to Patients. Edited by Norcross JC. London, Oxford University Press, 2002b, pp 129–143

Birmaher B, Brent DA, Kolko D, et al: Clinical outcome after short-term psychotherapy for adolescents with major depressive disorder. Arch Gen Psychiatry 57(1):29–36, 2000 10632230

Blodgett JC, Del Re AC, Maisel NC, Finney JW: A meta-analysis of topiramate's effects for individuals with alcohol use disorders. Alcohol Clin Exp Res 38(6):1481–1488, 2014 24796492

Bond M, Banon E, Grenier M: Differential effects of interventions on the therapeutic alliance with patients with personality disorders. J Psychother Pract Res 7(4):301–318, 1998 9752641

Bordin E: The generalizability of the psycho-analytic concept of the working alliance. Psychotherapy 16:252–260, 1979

Bormann JE, Thorp SR, Smith E, et al: Individual treatment of posttraumatic stress disorder using mantram repetition: a randomized clinical trial. Am J Psychiatry 175(10):979–988, 2018 29921143

Brenner AM: Teaching supportive psychotherapy in the twenty-first century. Harv Rev Psychiatry 20(5):259–267, 2012 23030214

Brent DA, Holder D, Kolko D, et al: A clinical psychotherapy trial for adolescent depression comparing cognitive, family, and supportive therapy. Arch Gen Psychiatry 54(9):877–885, 1997 9294380

Brill L: The treatment of drug abuse: evolution of a perspective. Am J Psychiatry 134(2):157–160, 1977 835736

Bronheim HE, Fulop G, Kunkel EJ, et al; The Academy of Psychosomatic Medicine: The Academy of Psychosomatic Medicine practice guidelines for psychiatric consultation in the general medical setting. Psychosomatics 39(4):S8–S30, 1998 9691717

Bryant RA, Sackville T, Dang ST, et al: Treating acute stress disorder: an evaluation of cognitive behavior therapy and supportive counseling techniques. Am J Psychiatry 156(11):1780–1786, 1999 10553743

Buckley P: Supportive therapy: a neglected treatment. Psychiatr Ann 16:515–521, 1986

Busch KA, Fawcett J, Jacobs DG: Clinical correlates of inpatient suicide. J Clin Psychiatry 64(1):14–19, 2003 12590618

Cailhol L, Rodgers R, Burnand Y, et al: Therapeutic alliance in short-term supportive and psychodynamic psychotherapies: a necessary but not sufficient condition for outcome? Psychiatry Res 170(2-3):229–233, 2009 19906442

Caplan G: An Approach to Community Mental Health. New York, Grune & Stratton, 1961

Carey KB, Cocco KM, Simons JS: Concurrent validity of clinicians' ratings of substance abuse among psychiatric outpatients. Psychiatr Serv 47(8):842–847, 1996 8837156

Carter FA, Jordan J, McIntosh VV, et al: The long-term efficacy of three psychotherapies for anorexia nervosa: a randomized, controlled trial. Int J Eat Disord 44(7):647–654, 2011 21997429

Chiles JA, Strosahl KD, Roberts LW: Clinical Manual for the Assessment and Treatment of Suicidal Patients, Second Edition. Washington, DC, American Psychiatric Association Publishing, 2019.

Clark DC, Fawcett J: A review of empirical risk factors for the evaluation of the suicidal patient, in The Assessment, Management, and Treatment of Suicide: Guidelines for Practice. Edited by Bongar B. New York, Oxford University Press, 1992, pp 16–48

Clarkin JF, Levy KN, Lenzenweger MF, Kernberg OF: Evaluating three treatments for borderline personality disorder: a multiwave study. Am J Psychiatry 164(6):922–928, 2007 17541052

Classen C, Butler LD, Koopman C, et al: Supportive-expressive group therapy and distress in patients with metastatic breast cancer: a randomized clinical intervention trial. Arch Gen Psychiatry 58(5):494–501, 2001 11343530

Clever SL, Tulsky JA: Dreaded conversations: moving beyond discomfort in patient-physician communication (editorial). J Gen Intern Med 17(11):884–885, 2002 12406362

Colby KM: A Primer for Psychotherapies. New York, Ronald Press, 1951

Cusack K, Jonas DE, Forneris CA, et al: Psychological treatments for adults with posttraumatic stress disorder: A systematic review and meta-analysis. Clin Psychol Rev 43:128–141, 2016 26574151

Davanloo H: A method of short-term dynamic psychotherapy, in Short-Term Dynamic Psychotherapy. Edited by Davanloo H. Northvale, NJ, Jason Aronson, 1980, pp 43–71

de Jonghe F, Rijnierse P, Janssen R: The role of support in psychoanalysis. J Am Psychoanal Assoc 40(2):475–499, 1992 1593081

de Maat S, Dekker J, Schoevers R, et al: Short psychodynamic supportive psycho-therapy, antidepressants, and their combination in the treatment of major de-pression: a mega-analysis based on three randomized clinical trials. Depress Anxiety 25(7):565–574, 2008 17557313

Dewald PA: The strategy of the therapeutic process, in Psychotherapy: A Dynamic Approach. New York, Basic Books, 1964, pp 95–108

Dewald PA: Psychotherapy: A Dynamic Approach, 2nd Edition. New York, Basic Books, 1971

Dewald PA: Principles of supportive psychotherapy. Am J Psychother 48(4):505–518, 1994 7872414

deWinstanley PA, Bjork RA: Successful lecturing: presenting information in ways that engage effective processing, in New Directions for Teaching and Learn-ing. Edited by Halpern D, Hakel M. San Francisco, CA, Jossey-Bass, 2002, pp 19–31

Douglas CJ: Teaching supportive psychotherapy to psychiatric residents. Am J Psychiatry 165(4):445–452, 2008 18381914

Drake RE, Sederer LI: Inpatient psychosocial treatment of chronic schizophrenia: negative effects and current guidelines. Hosp Community Psychiatry 37(9):897–901, 1986 3758971

Drake RE, McHugo GJ, Noordsy DL: Treatment of alcoholism among schizo-phrenic outpatients: 4-year outcomes. Am J Psychiatry 150(2):328–329, 1993 8422088

Drake RE, Essock SM, Shaner A, et al: Implementing dual diagnosis services for clients with severe mental illness. Psychiatr Serv 52(4):469–476, 2001 11274491

Driessen E, Smits N, Dekker JJ, et al: Differential efficacy of cognitive behavioral therapy and psychodynamic therapy for major depression: a study of prescriptive factors. Psychol Med 46(4):731–744, 2016 26750445

Dunn C, Deroo L, Rivara FP: The use of brief interventions adapted from motivational interviewing across behavioral domains: a systematic review. Addiction 96(12):1725–1742, 2001 11784466

Elkin I: The NIMH Treatment of Depression Collaborative Research Program: where we began and where we are, in Handbook of Psychotherapy and Behavioral Change. Edited by Bergin AE, Garfield SL. New York, Wiley, 1994, pp 114–139

Elkin I, Shea MT, Watkins JT, et al: National Institute of Mental Health Treatment of Depression Collaborative Research Program: general effectiveness of treatments. Arch Gen Psychiatry 46(11):971–982, discussion 983, 1989 2684085

Epstein RM, Hundert EM: Defining and assessing professional competence. JAMA 287(2):226–235, 2002 11779266

Evans S, Fishman B, Spielman L, Haley A: Randomized trial of cognitive behavior therapy versus supportive psychotherapy for HIV-related peripheral neuropathic pain. Psychosomatics 44(1):44–50, 2003 12515837

Everly GS Jr, Mitchell JT: Assisting Individuals in Crisis: A Workbook. Ellicott City, MD, International Critical Incident Stress Foundation, 1998

Everly GS Jr, Mitchell JT: Critical Incident Stress Management (CISM): A New Era and Standard of Care in Crisis Intervention, 2nd Edition. Ellicott City, MD, Chevron Publishing, 1999

Fawcett J, Scheftner WA, Fogg L, et al: Time-related predictors of suicide in major affective disorder. Am J Psychiatry 147(9):1189–1194, 1990 2104515

Fawcett J, Clark DC, Busch KA: Assessing and treating the patient at risk for suicide. Psychiatr Ann 23:244–255, 1993

Feinstein R, Heiman N, Yager J: Common factors affecting psychotherapy outcomes: some implications for teaching psychotherapy. J Psychiatr Pract 21(3):180–189, 2015 25955260

Fernandez-Pol B, Bluestone H, Mizruchi MS: Inner-city substance abuse patterns: a study of psychiatric inpatients. Am J Drug Alcohol Abuse 14(1):41–50, 1988 3265029

Fischer DE, Halikas JA, Baker JW, Smith JB: Frequency and patterns of drug abuse in psychiatric patients. Dis Nerv Syst 36(10):550–553, 1975 1164857

Foa EB: Trauma and women: course, predictors, and treatment. J Clin Psychiatry 58(suppl 9):25–28, 1997 9329448

Foa EB, Franklin ME: Psychotherapies for obsessive compulsive disorder: a review, in Obsessive Compulsive Disorder, 2nd Edition. Edited by Maj M, Sartorius N, Okasha A, et al. Chichester, UK, Wiley, 2002, pp 93–115

Foa EB, Rothbaum BO, Riggs DS, Murdock TB: Treatment of posttraumatic stress disorder in rape victims: a comparison between cognitive-behavioral procedures and counseling. J Consult Clin Psychol 59(5):715–723, 1991 1955605

Foa EB, Hembree EA, Cahill SP, et al: Randomized trial of prolonged exposure for posttraumatic stress disorder with and without cognitive restructuring: outcome at academic and community clinics. J Consult Clin Psychol 73(5):953–964, 2005 16287395

Fonagy P, Target M: Theoretical models of psychodynamic psychotherapy, in Textbook of Psychotherapeutic Treatments. Edited by Gabbard GO. Washington, DC, American Psychiatric Publishing, 2009, pp 3–42

Frank JB, Frank JD: Persuasion and Healing: A Comparison Study of Psychotherapy, 3rd Edition. Baltimore, MD, Johns Hopkins University Press, 1991

Frank JD: General psychotherapy: the restoration of morale, in American Handbook of Psychiatry, Vol 5: Treatment, 2nd Edition. Edited by Freedman DX, Dyrud JE. New York, Basic Books, 1975, pp 117–132

Frankl M, Philips B, Wennberg P: Psychotherapy role expectations and experiences: discrepancy and therapeutic alliance among patients with substance use disorders. Psychol Psychother 87(4):411–424, 2014 24415529

Freud S: The ego and the id (1923/1961), in The Standard Edition of the Complete Psychological Works of Sigmund Freud, Vol 19. Edited by Strachey J. London, Hogarth Press, 1961, pp 12–66

Freud S: Inhibitions, symptoms and anxiety (1926/1959), in The Standard Edition of the Complete Psychological Works of Sigmund Freud, Vol 20. Edited by Strachey J. London, Hogarth Press, 1959, pp 75–175

Friedman RS, Lister P: The current status of psychodynamic formulation. Psychiatry 50(2):126–141, 1987 3588773

Fudala PJ, Bridge TP, Herbert S, et al; Buprenorphine/Naloxone Collaborative Study Group: Office-based treatment of opiate addiction with a sublingual-tablet formulation of buprenorphine and naloxone. N Engl J Med 349(10):949–958, 2003 12954743

Fuller RK, Branchey L, Brightwell DR, et al: Disulfiram treatment of alcoholism: a Veterans Administration cooperative study. JAMA 256(11):1449–1455, 1986 3528541

Gabbard GO: A contemporary psychoanalytic model of countertransference. J Clin Psychol 57(8):983–991, 2001 11449380

Gabbard GO: Long-Term Psychodynamic Psychotherapy: A Basic Text, 3rd Edition. Washington, DC, American Psychiatric Publishing, 2017

Galanter M, Castaneda R, Ferman J: Substance abuse among general psychiatric patients: place of presentation, diagnosis, and treatment. Am J Drug Alcohol Abuse 14(2):211–235, 1988 3052039

Galynker G: The Suicidal Crisis: A Clinical Guide to the Assessment of Imminent Suicide Risk. New York, Oxford University Press, 2017

Gastelum E, Douglas CJ, Cabaniss DL: Teaching psychodynamic psychotherapy to psychiatric residents: an integrated approach. Psychodyn Psychiatry 41(1):127–140, 2013 23480164

Gaston L: The concept of the alliance and its role in psychotherapy: theoretical and empirical considerations. Psychotherapy 27:143–153, 1990

Gelso CJ, Fassinger RE, Gomez MJ, et al: Countertransference reactions to lesbian clients: the role of homophobia, counselor gender, and countertransference management. J Couns Psychol 42:356–364, 1995

Gelso CJ, Latts MG, Gomez MJ, Fassinger RE: Countertransference management and therapy outcome: an initial evaluation. J Clin Psychol 58(7):861–867, 2002 12205726

Gerstley L, McLellan AT, Alterman AI, et al: Ability to form an alliance with the therapist: a possible marker of prognosis for patients with antisocial personality disorder. Am J Psychiatry 146(4):508–512, 1989 2929752

Gill MM, Muslin HL: Early interpretation of transference. J Am Psychoanal Assoc 24(4):779–794, 1976 993562

Glass A: Psychotherapy in the combat zone. Am J Psychiatry 110:725–731, 1954

Glover E: The therapeutic effect of inexact interpretation: a contribution to the theory of suggestion. Int J Psychoanal 12:397–411, 1931

Glynn SM, Marder SR, Liberman RP, et al: Supplementing clinic-based skills training with manual-based community support sessions: effects on social adjustment of patients with schizophrenia. Am J Psychiatry 159(5):829–837, 2002 11986138

Goldberg RL, Green SA: A learning-theory perspective of brief psychodynamic psychotherapy. Am J Psychother 40(1):70–82, 1986 2870653

Goldman CR, Quinn FL: Effects of a patient education program in the treatment of schizophrenia. Hosp Community Psychiatry 39(3):282–286, 1988 3356434

Gorton GE: Psychodynamic approaches to the patient. Psychiatr Serv 51(11):1408–1409, 2000 11058188

Greenberg J: The analyst's participation: a new look. J Am Psychoanal Assoc 49(2):359–381, discussion 381–426, 2001 11508371

Greenson RR: The working alliance and the transference neurosis. Psychoanal Q 34:155–181, 1965 14302976

Greenson RR: The Technique and Practice of Psychoanalysis. New York, International Universities Press, 1967, pp 190–216

Gunderson JG, Frank AF, Katz HM, et al: Effects of psychotherapy in schizophrenia, II: comparative outcome of two forms of treatment. Schizophr Bull 10(4):564–598, 1984 6151246

Harder S, Koester A, Valbak K, et al: Five year follow-up of supportive psychodynamic psychotherapy in first-episode psychosis: long-term outcome in social functioning. Psychiatry 77(2):155–168, 2014 24865198

Hartley DE, Strupp HH: The therapeutic alliance: its relationship to outcome in brief psychotherapy, in Empirical Studies of Psychoanalytical Theories, Vol 1. Edited by Masling J. Hillsdale, NJ, Analytic Press, 1983, pp 1–27

Hartmann H: Ego Psychology and the Problem of Adaptation (1939/1958). Translated by Rapaport D. New York, International Universities Press, 1958

Hasin DS, Grant BF: The National Epidemiologic Survey on Alcohol and Related Conditions (NESARC) Waves 1 and 2: review and summary of findings. Soc Psychiatry Psychiatr Epidemiol 50(11):1609–1640, 2015 26210739

Hawton K: Assessment of suicide risk. Br J Psychiatry 150:145–153, 1987 3307975

Heinssen RK, Liberman RP, Kopelowicz A: Psychosocial skills training for schizophrenia: lessons from the laboratory. Schizophr Bull 26(1):21–46, 2000 10755668

Hellerstein DJ, Pinsker H, Rosenthal RN, Klee S: Supportive therapy as the treatment model of choice. J Psychother Pract Res 3(4):300–306, 1994 22700197

Hellerstein DJ, Rosenthal RN, Miner CR: A prospective study of integrated outpatient treatment for substance-abusing schizophrenia patients. Am J Addict 4:33–42, 1995

Hellerstein DJ, Rosenthal RN, Pinsker H, et al: A randomized prospective study comparing supportive and dynamic therapies: outcome and alliance. J Psychother Pract Res 7(4):261–271, 1998 9752637

Hellerstein DJ, Kocsis JH, Chapman D, et al: Double-blind comparison of sertraline, imipramine, and placebo in the treatment of dysthymia: effects on personality. Am J Psychiatry 157(9):1436–1444, 2000 10964860

Henry WP, Schacht TE, Strupp HH: Structural analysis of social behavior: application to a study of interpersonal process in differential psychotherapeutic outcome. J Consult Clin Psychol 54(1):27–31, 1986 3958298

Henry WP, Schacht TE, Strupp HH: Patient and therapist introject, interpersonal process, and differential psychotherapy outcome. J Consult Clin Psychol 58(6):768–774, 1990 2292626

Herbert JD, Gaudiano BA, Rheingold AA, et al: Cognitive behavior therapy for generalized social anxiety disorder in adolescents: a randomized controlled trial. J Anxiety Disord 23(2):167–177, 2009 18653310

Ho AP, Tsuang JW, Liberman RP, et al: Achieving effective treatment of patients with chronic psychotic illness and comorbid substance dependence. Am J Psychiatry 156(11):1765–1770, 1999 10553741

Hogarty GE, Kornblith SJ, Greenwald D, et al: Three-year trials of personal therapy among schizophrenic patients living with or independent of family, I: description of study and effects on relapse rates. Am J Psychiatry 154(11):1504–1513, 1997 9356557

Holmes J: Supportive psychotherapy: the search for positive meanings. Br J Psychiatry 167(4):439–445, discussion 446–447, 1995 8829709

Horowitz M, Marmar C: The therapeutic alliance with difficult patients, in Psychiatry Update: The American Psychiatric Association Annual Review, Vol 4. Edited by Hales RE, Frances AJ. Washington, DC, American Psychiatric Press, 1985, pp 573–585

Horowitz MJ, Marmar C, Weiss DS, et al: Brief psychotherapy of bereavement reactions: the relationship of process to outcome. Arch Gen Psychiatry 41(5):438–448, 1984 6721669

Horvath AO, Symonds BD: Relation between working alliance and outcome in psychotherapy: a meta-analysis. J Couns Psychol 38:139–149, 1991

Horvath AO, Del Re AC, Flückiger C, Symonds D: Alliance in individual psychotherapy. Psychotherapy (Chic) 48(1):9–16, 2011 21401269

Hunter J, Leszcz M, McLachlan SA, et al: Psychological stress response in breast cancer. Psychooncology 5:4–14, 1996

Imber SD, Pilkonis PA, Sotsky SM, et al: Mode-specific effects among three treatments for depression. J Consult Clin Psychol 58(3):352–359, 1990 2195085

James RK, Gilliland BE: Crisis Intervention Strategies, 4th Edition. Belmont, CA, Brooks/Cole Thomson Learning, 2001

Jellinek EM: Phases of alcohol addiction. Q J Stud Alcohol 13(4):673–684, 1952 13014274

Joiner TE: Why People Die by Suicide. Cambridge, MA: Harvard University Press, 2005

Jørgensen CR, Freund C, Bøye R, et al: Outcome of mentalization-based and supportive psychotherapy in patients with borderline personality disorder: a randomized trial. Acta Psychiatr Scand 127(4):305–317, 2013 22897123

Kates J, Rockland LH: Supportive psychotherapy of the schizophrenic patient. Am J Psychother 48(4):543–561, 1994 7872417

Kaufman ER: Countertransference and other mutually interactive aspects of psychotherapy with substance abusers. Am J Addict 1:185–202, 1992

Kaufman E, Reoux J: Guidelines for the successful psychotherapy of substance abusers. Am J Drug Alcohol Abuse 14(2):199–209, 1988 3177339

Keller DS, Carroll KM, Nick C, et al: Differential treatment response in alexithymic cocaine abusers: findings from a randomized clinical trial of psychotherapy and pharmacotherapy. Am J Addict 4:234–244, 1995

Kessler RC, McGonagle KA, Zhao S, et al: Lifetime and 12-month prevalence of DSM-III-R psychiatric disorders in the United States: results from the National Comorbidity Survey. Arch Gen Psychiatry 51(1):8–19, 1994 8279933

Khantzian EJ: The self-medication hypothesis of addictive disorders: focus on heroin and cocaine dependence. Am J Psychiatry 142(11):1259–1264, 1985 3904487

Kiesler DJ: Therapist countertransference: in search of common themes and empirical referents. J Clin Psychol 57(8):1053–1063, 2001 11449388

Kleber HD: Pharmacologic treatments for heroin and cocaine dependence. Am J Addict 12(suppl s2):S5–S18, 2003 12857659

Klein DF, Zitrin CM, Woerner MG, Ross DC: Treatment of phobias, II: behavior therapy and supportive psychotherapy: are there any specific ingredients? Arch Gen Psychiatry 40(2):139–145, 1983 6130751

Kocsis JH, Gelenberg AJ, Rothbaum BO, et al; REVAMP Investigators: Cognitive behavioral analysis system of psychotherapy and brief supportive psychotherapy for augmentation of antidepressant nonresponse in chronic depression: the REVAMP trial. Arch Gen Psychiatry 66(11):1178–1188, 2009 19884606

Kool S, Dekker J, Duijsens IJ, et al: Changes in personality pathology after pharmacotherapy and combined therapy for depressed patients. J Pers Disord 17(1):60–72, 2003 12659547

Koss M, Shiang J: Research on brief psychotherapy, in Handbook of Psychotherapy and Behavior Change. Edited by Bergin A, Garfield S. New York, John Wiley, 1994, pp 664–700

Kozart MF: Understanding efficacy in psychotherapy: an ethnomethodological perspective on the therapeutic alliance. Am J Orthopsychiatry 72(2):217–231, 2002 15792061

Lamberti JS, Herz MI: Psychotherapy, social skills training, and vocational rehabilitation in schizophrenia, in Contemporary Issues in the Treatment of Schizophrenia. Edited by Shriqui CL, Nasrallah HA. Washington, DC, American Psychiatric Press, 1995, pp 713–734

Lauriello J, Bustillo J, Keith SJ: A critical review of research on psychosocial treatment of schizophrenia. Biol Psychiatry 46(10):1409–1417, 1999 10578455

Lecomte T, Liberman RP, Wallace CJ: Identifying and using reinforcers to enhance the treatment of persons with serious mental illness. Psychiatr Serv 51(10):1312–1314, 2000 11013335

le Grange D, Crosby RD, Rathouz PJ, Leventhal BL: A randomized controlled comparison of family-based treatment and supportive psychotherapy for adolescent bulimia nervosa. Arch Gen Psychiatry 64(9):1049–1056, 2007 17768270

Lehman AF, Herron JD, Schwartz RP, Myers CP: Rehabilitation for adults with severe mental illness and substance use disorders: a clinical trial. J Nerv Ment Dis 181(2):86–90, 1993 8426176

Lewis G, Appleby L: Personality disorder: the patients psychiatrists dislike. Br J Psychiatry 153:44–49, 1988 3224249

Liberman RP, Wallace CJ, Blackwell G, et al: Skills training versus psychosocial occupational therapy for persons with persistent schizophrenia. Am J Psychiatry 155(8):1087–1091, 1998 9699698

Lindemann E: Symptomatology and management of acute grief 1944. Am J Psychiatry 151(6 suppl):155–1608, 1994 8192191

Linehan MM: Cognitive-Behavioral Treatment of Borderline Personality Disorder. New York, Guilford, 1993

Linehan MM, Tutek DA, Heard HL, Armstrong HE: Interpersonal outcome of cognitive behavioral treatment for chronically suicidal borderline patients. Am J Psychiatry 151(12):1771–1776, 1994 7977884

Lipsitz JD, Gur M, Vermes D, et al: A randomized trial of interpersonal therapy versus supportive therapy for social anxiety disorder. Depress Anxiety 25(6):542–553, 2008 17941096

Luborsky L: Principles of Psychoanalytic Psychotherapy: A Manual for Supportive-Expressive Treatment. New York, Basic Books, 1984

Luborsky L, Crits-Christoph P: Understanding Transference: The Core Conflictual Relationship Theme Method. New York, Basic Books, 1990

Luborsky L, Mark D: Short-term supportive-expressive psychoanalytic psychotherapy, in Handbook of Short-Term Dynamic Psychotherapy. Edited by Crits-Christoph P, Barber JP. New York, Basic Books, 1991, pp 110–136

Lysaker PH, Kukla M, Belanger E, et al: Individual psychotherapy and changes in self-experience in schizophrenia: a qualitative comparison of patients in metacognitively focused and supportive psychotherapy. Psychiatry 78(4):305–316, 2015 26745684

Maina G, Forner F, Bogetto F: Randomized controlled trial comparing brief dynamic and supportive therapy with waiting list condition in minor depressive disorders. Psychother Psychosom 74(1):43–50, 2005 15627856

Malan DH: Individual Psychotherapy and the Science of Psychodynamics. London, Butterworth, 1979

Manring J, Beitman BD, Dewan MJ: Evaluating competence in psychotherapy. Paper presented at the Annual Meeting of the American Psychiatric Association, San Francisco, CA, May 2003

Markowitz JC, Klerman GL, Clougherty KF, et al: Individual psychotherapies for depressed HIV-positive patients. Am J Psychiatry 152(10):1504–1509, 1995 7573591

Markowitz JC, Petkova E, Neria Y, et al: Is exposure necessary? A randomized clinical trial of interpersonal psychotherapy for PTSD. Am J Psychiatry 172(5):430–440, 2015 25677355

Marlatt GA, Gordon JR: Determinants of relapse: implications for the maintenance of behavior change, in Behavioral Medicine: Changing Health Lifestyles. Edited by Davidson PO, Davidson SM. New York, Brunner/Mazel, 1980, pp 410–452

Marlatt GA, Gordon JR: Relapse Prevention: Maintenance Strategies in the Treatment of Addictive Behaviors. New York, Guilford, 1985

Massie MJ, Holland JC: Depression and the cancer patient. J Clin Psychiatry 51(suppl):12–17, discussion 18–19, 1990 2195008

McGorry PD, Nelson B, Phillips LJ, et al: Randomized controlled trial of interventions for young people at ultra-high risk of psychosis: twelve-month outcome. J Clin Psychiatry 74(4):349–356, 2013 23218022

Menninger K: Theory of Psychoanalytic Technique. London, Imago, 1958

Messer SB: A psychodynamic perspective on resistance in psychotherapy: vive la résistance. J Clin Psychol 58(2):157–163, 2002 11793328

Mezirow J: On critical reflection. Adult Educ Q 48:185–198, 1998

Miller WR, Rollnick S: Motivational Interviewing: Preparing People to Change Addictive Behavior. New York, Guilford, 1991

Miller WR, Rose GS: Motivational interviewing in relational context. Am Psychol 65:298–299, 2010

Misch DA: Basic strategies of dynamic supportive therapy. J Psychother Pract Res 9(4):173–189, 2000 11069130

Mitchell JT, Everly GS Jr: Critical Incident Stress Debriefing (CISD): An Operations Manual for the Prevention of Traumatic Stress Among Emergency Service and Disaster Workers, 2nd Edition. Ellicott City, MD, Chevron, 1996

Mitchell JT, Everly GS Jr: Critical Incident Stress Management (CISM): Basic Group Crisis Intervention, 3rd Edition. Ellicott City, MD, International Critical Incident Stress Foundation, 2003

Mitchell SA: Relational Concepts in Psychoanalysis: An Integration. Cambridge, MA, Harvard University Press, 1988

Mumford E, Schlesinger HJ, Glass GV: The effect of psychological intervention on recovery from surgery and heart attacks: an analysis of the literature. Am J Public Health 72(2):141–151, 1982 7055315

Novalis PN, Rojcewicz J, Peele R: Clinical Manual of Supportive Psychotherapy. Washington, DC, American Psychiatric Association Publishing, 1993

Novalis PN, Singer V, Peele R: Clinical Manual of Supportive Psychotherapy. Washington, DC, American Psychiatric Association Publishing, 2020

Nunberg H: The synthetic function of the ego. Int J Psychoanal 12:123–140, 1931

Okuyama T, Akechi T, Mackenzie L, Furukawa TA: Psychotherapy for depression among advanced, incurable cancer patients: a systematic review and meta-analysis. Cancer Treat Rev 56:16–27, 2017 28453966

O'Malley SS, Jaffe AJ, Chang G, et al: Naltrexone and coping skills therapy for alcohol dependence: a controlled study. Arch Gen Psychiatry 49(11):881–887, 1992 1444726

Othmer E, Othmer S: The Clinical Interview Using DSM-IV, Vol 1. Washington, DC, American Psychiatric Press, 1994, pp 87–97

Palmer RL: Dialectical behavior therapy for borderline personality disorder. Adv Psychiatr Treat 8:10–16, 2002

Parad HJ, Parad LG: Crisis Intervention, Book 2: The Practitioner's Sourcebook for Brief Therapy. Milwaukee, WI, Family Service America, 1990

Parloff MB: Goals in psychotherapy: mediating and ultimate, in Goals of Psychotherapy. Edited by Mahrer AR. New York, Appleton-Century-Crofts, 1967, pp 5–19

Perry JC, Banon E, Ianni F: Effectiveness of psychotherapy for personality disorders. Am J Psychiatry 156(9):1312–1321, 1999 10484939

Perry S, Cooper AM, Michels R: The psychodynamic formulation: its purpose, structure, and clinical application. Am J Psychiatry 144(5):543–550, 1987 3578562

Persons JB: Cognitive Therapy in Practice: A Case Formulation Approach. New York, WW Norton, 1989

Persons JB: Case conceptualization in cognitive-behavior therapy, in Cognitive Therapies in Action: Evolving Innovative Practice. Edited by Kuehlwein KT, Rosen H. San Francisco, CA, Jossey-Bass, 1993, pp 33–53

Peselow ED, Sanfilipo MP, Fieve RR, Gulbenkian G: Personality traits during depression and after clinical recovery. Br J Psychiatry 164(3):349–354, 1994 8199788

Pine F: The interpretive moment: variations on classical themes. Bull Menninger Clin 48(1):54–71, 1984 6692050

Pinsker H: A Primer of Supportive Psychotherapy. Hillsdale, NJ, Analytic Press, 1997

Pinsker H, Rosenthal RN: Beth Israel Medical Center Supportive Psychotherapy Manual (Social and Behavioral Sciences Documents, Vol 18, No 2). New York, Beth Israel Medical Center, 1988

Pinsker H, Rosenthal R, McCullough L: Dynamic supportive psychotherapy, in Handbook of Short-Term Dynamic Psychotherapy. Edited by Crits-Christoph P, Barber JP. New York, Basic Books, 1991, pp 220–247

Pinsker H, Hellerstein DJ, Rosenthal RN, et al: Supportive therapy, common factors and eclecticism. Paper presented at the Annual Meeting of the American Psychiatric Association, New York, May 1996

Pinsker H, Mellman L, Beresin E, et al: AADPRT Supportive Therapy Competencies. Lebanon, PA, American Association of Directors of Psychiatric Residency Training, November 2001

Piper WE, Joyce AS, McCallum M, Azim HF: Interpretive and supportive forms of psychotherapy and patient personality variables. J Consult Clin Psychol 66(3):558–567, 1998 9642895

Pokorny AD: Prediction of suicide in psychiatric patients: report of a prospective study. Arch Gen Psychiatry 40(3):249–257, 1983 6830404

Pollack J, Flegenheimer W, Winston A: Brief adaptive psychotherapy, in Handbook of Short-Term Dynamic Psychotherapy. Edited by Crits-Christoph P, Barber JP. New York, Basic Books, 1991, pp 199–219

Posner K, Brent D, Lucas C, et al: Columbia-Suicide Severity Rating Scale (C-SSRS). New York, Columbia University/New York State Psychiatric Institute, 2009

Prochaska JO, DiClemente CC: The Transtheoretical Approach: Crossing Traditional Boundaries of Therapy. Homewood, IL, Dow Jones-Irwin, 1984

Psychopathology Committee of the Group for the Advancement of Psychiatry: Reexamination of therapist self-disclosure. Psychiatr Serv 52(11):1489–1493, 2001 11684745

Puryear DA: Helping People in Crisis. San Francisco, CA, Jossey-Bass, 1979

Quality Assurance Project: Treatment outlines for the management of the somatoform disorders. Aust N Z J Psychiatry 19(4):397–407, 1985 3869006

Rea MM, Strachan AM, Goldstein MJ, et al: Changes in patient coping style following individual and family treatment for schizophrenia. Br J Psychiatry 158:642–647, 1991 1860018

Regier DA, Farmer ME, Rae DS, et al: Comorbidity of mental disorders with alcohol and other drug abuse: results from the Epidemiologic Catchment Area (ECA) Study. JAMA 264(19):2511–2518, 1990 2232018

Renaud J, Brent DA, Baugher M, et al: Rapid response to psychosocial treatment for adolescent depression: a two-year follow-up. J Am Acad Child Adolesc Psychiatry 37(11):1184–1190, 1998 9808930

Richard ML, Liskow BI, Perry PJ: Recent psychostimulant use in hospitalized schizophrenics. J Clin Psychiatry 46(3):79–83, 1985 2857708

Robbins B: Under attack: devaluation and the challenge of tolerating the transference. J Psychother Pract Res 9(3):136–141, 2000 10896738

Roberts AR: An overview of crisis theory and crisis intervention, in Crisis Intervention Handbook. Edited by Roberts AR. New York, Oxford University Press, 2000, pp 3–30

Roberts LW: A Clinical Guide to Psychiatric Ethics. Arlington, VA, American Psychiatric Association Publishing, 2016

Rockland LH: Supportive Therapy: A Psychodynamic Approach. New York, Basic Books, 1989

Rollnick S, Miller WR: What is motivational interviewing? Behav Cogn Psychother 23:325–334, 1995

Rosenbaum B, Harder S, Knudsen P, et al: Supportive psychodynamic psychotherapy versus treatment as usual for first-episode psychosis: two-year outcome. Psychiatry 75(4):331–341, 2012 23244011

Rosenthal RN: Group treatments for schizophrenic substance abusers, in The Group Therapy of Substance Abuse. Edited by Brook DW, Spitz HI. New York, Haworth Medical Press, 2002, pp 329–351

Rosenthal RN: Techniques of individual supportive psychotherapy, in Textbook of Psychotherapeutic Treatments. Edited by Gabbard GO. Washington, DC, American Psychiatric Publishing, 2009, pp 417–445

Rosenthal RN, Westreich L: Treatment of persons with dual diagnoses of substance use disorder and other psychological problems, in Addictions: A Comprehensive Guidebook. Edited by McCrady GA, Epstein EE. New York, Oxford University Press, 1999, pp 439–476

Rosenthal RN, Muran JC, Pinsker H, et al: Interpersonal change in brief supportive psychotherapy. J Psychother Pract Res 8(1):55–63, 1999 9888107

Rosenthal RN, Miner CR, Sena P, et al: The therapeutic alliance in group treatments for substance pabusers with schizophrenia. Paper Presented at the Annual Meeting of the American Psychiatric Association, Chicago, IL, May 2000

Rosenzweig S: Some implicit common factors in diverse methods of psychotherapy. Am J Orthopsychiatry 6:412–415, 1936

Rounsaville BJ, Carroll KM: Individual psychotherapy, in Principles of Addiction Medicine. Edited by Graham AW, Schultz TK. Chevy Chase, MD, American Society of Addiction Medicine, 1998, pp 631–652

Sachse R, Kramer U: Clarification-oriented psychotherapy of dependent personality disorder. J Contemp Psychother 48:1–11, 2018

Safran JD, Muran JC: Negotiating the Therapeutic Alliance: A Relational Treatment Guide. New York, Guilford, 2000, pp 6–12

Salmon TW: War neuroses and their lesson. New York Medical Journal 59:993–994, 1919

Sampson H, Weiss J: Testing hypotheses: the approach of the Mount Zion Psychotherapy Research Group, in The Psychotherapeutic Process: A Research Handbook. Edited by Greenberg LS, Pinsof WM. New York, Guilford, 1986, pp 591–613

Sandoval J: Crisis counseling: conceptualizations and genetic principles. School Psych Rev 14:257–265, 1985

Scaturo DJ: A tripartite learning conceptualization of psychotherapy: the therapeutic alliance, technical interventions, and relearning. Am J Psychother 64(1):1–27, 2010 20405762

Schramm E, Kriston L, Zobel I, et al: Effect of disorder-specific vs nonspecific psychotherapy for chronic depression: A randomized clinical trial. JAMA Psychiatry 74(3):233–242, 2017 28146251

Sharf J, Primavera LH, Diener MJ: Dropout and therapeutic alliance: a meta-analysis of adult individual psychotherapy. Psychotherapy (Chic) 47(4):637–645, 2010 21198249

Shear MK, Houck P, Greeno C, Masters S: Emotion-focused psychotherapy for patients with panic disorder. Am J Psychiatry 158(12):1993–1998, 2001 11729015

Sifneos PE: The prevalence of 'alexithymic' characteristics in psychosomatic patients. Psychother Psychosom 22(2):255–262, 1973 4770536

Sifneos PE: Problems of psychotherapy of patients with alexithymic characteristics and physical disease. Psychother Psychosom 26(2):65–70, 1975 1202547

Simon JC: Criteria for therapist self-disclosure. Am J Psychother 42(3):404–415, 1988 3177704

Skaikeu KA: Crisis Intervention. Boston, Allyn & Bacon, 1990

Smith TE, Hull JW, Goodman M, et al: The relative influences of symptoms, insight, and neurocognition on social adjustment in schizophrenia and schizoaffective disorder. J Nerv Ment Dis 187(2):102–108, 1999 10067950

Spiegel D, Classen C: Acute stress disorders, in Treatments of Psychiatric Disorders, 2nd Edition. Edited by Gabbard GO. Washington, DC, American Psychiatric Press, 1995, pp 1521–1536

Stanton AH, Gunderson JG, Knapp PH, et al: Effects of psychotherapy in schizophrenia, I: design and implementation of a controlled study. Schizophr Bull 10(4):520–563, 1984 6151245

Sudak DM, Goldberg DA: Trends in psychotherapy training: a national survey of psychiatry residency training. Acad Psychiatry 36(5):369–373, 2012 22983467

Thomas EM, Weiss SM: Nonpharmacological interventions with chronic cancer pain in adults. Cancer Contr 7(2):157–164, 2000 10783820

Thompson LW, Gallagher D: Depression and its treatment. Aging (Milano) 348:14–18, 1985

Tompkins MA: Cognitive-behavioral case formulation: the case of Jim. J Psychother Integration 6:97–105, 1996

Truong A, Wu P, Diez-Barroso R, Coverdale J: What is the efficacy of teaching psychotherapy to psychiatry residents and medical students? Acad Psychiatry 39(5):575–579, 2015 25933647

Ursano RJ, Silberman EK: Psychoanalysis, psychoanalytic psychotherapy, and supportive psychotherapy, in The American Psychiatric Press Textbook of Psychiatry, 3rd Edition. Edited by Hales RE, Yudofsky SC, Talbott JA. Washington, DC, 1999, pp 1157–1183

Vaillant GE: Adaptation to Life. Boston, MA, Little, Brown, 1977

Vaillant GE (ed): Empirical Studies of Ego Mechanisms of Defense. Washington, DC, American Psychiatric Press, 1986

van der Kolk BA, Spinazzola J, Blaustein ME, et al: A randomized clinical trial of eye movement desensitization and reprocessing (EMDR), fluoxetine, and pill placebo in the treatment of posttraumatic stress disorder: treatment effects and long-term maintenance. J Clin Psychiatry 68(1):37–46, 2007 17284128 van Emmerik AAP, Kamphuis JH, Hulsbosch AM, Emmelkamp PM: Single session debriefing after psychological trauma: a meta-analysis. Lancet 360(9335):766–771, 2002 12241834

van Gelderen MJ, Nijdam MJ, Vermetten E: An innovative framework for delivering psychotherapy to patients with treatment-resistant posttraumatic stress disorder: rationale for interactive motion-assisted therapy. Front Psychiatry 9:176, 2018 29780334

Vaughn CE, Leff JP: The influence of family and social factors on the course of psychiatric illness: a comparison of schizophrenic and depressed neurotic patients. Br J Psychiatry 129:125–137, 1976 963348

Viederman M: A model for interpretative supportive dynamic psychotherapy. Psychiatry 71(4):349–358, 2008 19152284

Vinnars B, Barber JP, Norén K, et al: Manualized supportive-expressive psychotherapy versus nonmanualized community-delivered psychodynamic therapy for patients with personality disorders: bridging efficacy and effectiveness. Am J Psychiatry 162(10):1933–1940, 2005 16199841

Volpicelli JR, Alterman AI, Hayashida M, O'Brien CP: Naltrexone in the treatment of alcohol dependence. Arch Gen Psychiatry 49(11):876–880, 1992 1345133

Wachtel P: Therapeutic Communication: Principles and Effective Practice. New York, Guilford, 1993

Wallerstein RS: Forty-Two Lives in Treatment: A Study of Psychoanalysis and Psychotherapy. New York, Guilford, 1986

Wallerstein RS: The psychotherapy research project of the Menninger Foundation: an overview. J Consult Clin Psychol 57(2):195–205, 1989 2708605

Walsh BT, Wilson GT, Loeb KL, et al: Medication and psychotherapy in the treatment of bulimia nervosa. Am J Psychiatry 154(4):523–531, 1997 9090340

Waltz J, Addis ME, Koerner K, Jacobson NS: Testing the integrity of a psychotherapy protocol: assessment of adherence and competence. J Consult Clin Psychol 61(4):620–630, 1993 8370857

Werman DS: The Practice of Supportive Psychotherapy. New York, Brunner/Mazel, 1984

Westerman MA, Foote JP, Winston A: Change in coordination across phases of psychotherapy and outcome: two mechanisms for the role played by patients' contribution to the alliance. J Consult Clin Psychol 63(4):672–675, 1995 7673546

Wilhelm S, Deckersbach T, Coffey BJ, et al: Habit reversal versus supportive psychotherapy for Tourette's disorder: a randomized controlled trial. Am J Psychiatry 160(6):1175–1177, 2003 12777279

Wilkinson CB, Vera E: Management and treatment of disaster victims. Psychiatr Ann 15:174–184, 1985

Winnicott DW: The Maturational Process and the Facilitating Environment: Studies in the Theory of Emotional Development. London, Hogarth, 1965

Winston A, Winston B: Handbook of Integrated Short-Term Psychotherapy. Washington, DC, American Psychiatric Publishing, 2002

Winston A, Pinsker H, McCullough L: A review of supportive psychotherapy. Hosp Community Psychiatry 37(11):1105–1114, 1986 3781499

Winston A, Rosenthal RN, Muran JC: Supportive psychotherapy, in Handbook of Personality Disorders: Theory, Research, and Treatment. Edited by Livesley WJ. New York, Guilford, 2001, pp 344–358

Woody GE, McLellan AT, Luborsky L, O'Brien CP: Sociopathy and psychotherapy outcome. Arch Gen Psychiatry 42(11):1081–1086, 1985 4051686

Yrondi A, Rieu J, Massip C, et al: Depressed patients' preferences for type of psychotherapy: a preliminary study. Patient Prefer Adherence 9:1371–1374, 2015 26491265

Zetzel ER: Current concepts of transference. Int J Psychoanal 37(4-5):369–376, 1956 13366506

Ziedonis D, Fisher W: Motivation-based assessment and treatment of substance abuse in patients with schizophrenia. Dir Psychiatry 16:1–7, 1996

Ziedonis DM, Trudeau K: Motivation to quit using substances among individuals with schizophrenia: implications for a motivation-based treatment model. Schizophr Bull 23(2):229–238, 1997 9165633

Zitrin CM, Klein DF, Woerner MG: Behavior therapy, supportive psychotherapy, imipramine, and phobias. Arch Gen Psychiatry 35(3):307–316, 1978 31847

Index

Page numbers printed in **boldface** *type refer to tables or figures.*

Help-rejecting, as contraindication
for supportive psychotherapy, 94
HIV-positive patients, and depression,
92
Holding environment, and anxiety
reduction, 66
Homeostasis, and crisis intervention,
122
Hospitalization, of suicidal patients,
135

Ideals, and case formulation, 45
Imipramine, 175, 176
Impulse control, and case formulation,
44
Initiation, of supportive psychotherapy,
95. *See also* Beginning phase
Integrated psychotherapy, for PTSD,
133
Interpersonal communication theory,
and countertransference, 118–119
Interpersonal relationships. *See also*
Family; Friends
professional boundaries and, 103
therapeutic alliance and, 55–56
Interpersonal therapy
for eating disorders, 177
for PTSD, 133
for social anxiety disorder, 176
Interpretation
expressive approach to transference
and, 108–109
techniques of supportive psychotherapy and, 70–71
Interpretive psychotherapy, for
personality disorders, 176
Interventions. *See also* Crisis intervention; Techniques
specific techniques, 53
transferences as guides to, 106
Inventory of Interpersonal Problems,
176

Lateness, of patients for sessions, 96–97
Learning theory, 28–29

Lending ego, 64
Limit setting, and conduct of sessions,
98
Long-term psychotherapy, indications
for, 101
Loss, and crisis intervention, 122

Major depression
contraindications for supportive
psychotherapy and, 94
outcome research on supportive
psychotherapy for, 175
video vignette of misalliance and,
111–113
Maladaptive behavior
countertransference and patterns of,
117–118
psychodynamically oriented therapy
and, 26
Malingering, 94
Mania, 143
Maxims, and normalizing, 60
Medical illness. *See also* Cancer
indications for supportive psychotherapy and, 92
outcome research on supportive
psychotherapy for, 177
Medications. *See also* Self-medication
personality disorders and, 148
substance use disorders and, 151
suicidal patients and, 135
Menninger psychotherapy research
project, 27, 89, 172–173
Mental illness. *See also* Anxiety
disorders; Bipolar disorder; Co-
occurring mental disorders;
Depression; Personality disorders;
Posttraumatic stress disorder;
Psychopathology; Psychotic
disorders
indications for supportive psychotherapy and chronic,
93–94
supportive psychotherapy for
severe forms of, 141–142